Rationing of health care in medicine

Papers based on a conference organised by the Royal College of Physicians and The Institute of Health Services Management

Edited by

Michael Tunbridge
Consultant Physician
Newcastle General Hospital

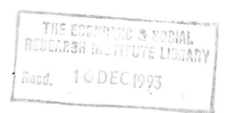

362.1

1993

ROYAL COLLEGE OF PHYSICIANS OF LONDON

Royal College of Physicians of London
11 St Andrews Place, London NW1 4LE

Registered Charity No. 210508

Copyright © 1993 Royal College of Physicians of London
ISBN 1 873240 59 7

Typeset by Dan-Set Graphics, Telford, Shropshire
Printed in Great Britain by Cathedral Print Services Ltd,
Rollestone Street, Salisbury SP1 1DX

Foreword

by Leslie Turnberg
President, Royal College of Physicians

There have always been limits on the provision of health care in every society and it is for society to set the boundaries which it finds acceptable. They may be defined in terms of available cash, quality and quantity of care, scientific and human considerations. The principle that there is a need for some form of priority setting is relatively clear and widely accepted within the health service but members of the public still largely expect that the service will provide whatever care is necessary for their nearest and dearest whenever required. Practising clinicians, particularly at the acute end of the spectrum of health care, point to the difficulties of meeting those demands in an open-ended service with restricted resources. The moral and ethical dilemmas faced by individual doctors facing individual patients cannot be ignored. Economic restraints may limit the availability of new techniques or the introduction of new drugs, but quite reasonably this leads to questions about the value of both new and old forms of treatment. Facing up to the choices involved means making difficult decisions and being responsible for the consequences. Both purchasers and providers need to be able to make informed choices based on high standards which can or should be achievable. It is the responsibility of the medical profession to develop the clinical measures which may be valuable in reaching informed decisions, but it is the wider constituency of the public through Government that makes the decisions to allocate resources.

The conference at which the papers in this book were presented took place in November 1992 under the auspices of the Royal College of Physicians and the Institute of Health Services Management. It was designed to involve doctors and managers in addressing some of the issues of rationing as applied to clinical medicine and in exploring the process by which decisions are reached. It is to be hoped that the publication of such thought provoking papers will lead to better understanding and wider debate of these important issues which cannot be ignored.

Finally, I am grateful to Professor Michael Peckham and Professor Sir Bernard Tomlinson for having presided over the sessions on 'Rationing in practice' and 'Facing up to the choices' respectively, and to Dr Michael Tunbridge for his thoughtful planning of a valuable and timely conference.

L.T.

Contributors

K C Calman, *Chief Medical Officer, Department of Health, Richmond House, 79 Whitehall, London SW1A 2NS.*

J Grimley Evans, *Professor of Geriatric Medicine, Department of Clinical Geratology, Radcliffe Infirmary, Oxford OX2 6HE.*

J B L Howell, *Chairman, Southampton & South West Hampshire Health Authority, Western Hospital, Oakley Road, Millbrook, Southampton SO9 4WQ.*

E P Kirk, *Chairman, Department of Obstetrics and Gynecology, Oregon Health Sciences University, 3181 SW Sam Jackson Park Road, Portland, Oregon 97201-3098, USA.*

R Klein, *Director, Centre for the Analysis of Social Policy, School of Social Sciences, University of Bath, Claverton Down, Bath BA2 7AY.*

N P Mallick, *Professor of Renal Medicine, Department of Renal and General Medicine, Manchester Royal Infirmary, Oxford Road, Manchester M13 9WL.*

A Maynard, *Director, Centre for Health Economics, University of York, Heslington, York YO1 5DD.*

R M Nicholls, *Executive Director, London Implementation Group, NHS Management Executive, Department of Health, 13–16 Russell Square, London WC1B 5EP.*

M D Rawlins, *Professor of Clinical Pharmacology, Wolfson Unit of Clinical Pharmacology, University of Newcastle, Newcastle upon Tyne NE2 4HH.*

W M G Tunbridge, *Consultant Physician, Newcastle General Hospital, Westgate Road, Newcastle upon Tyne NE4 6BE.*

Contents

Part 3: FACING UP TO THE CHOICES

1 | The economics of rationing health care

Alan Maynard

Professor of Economics and Director of the
Centre for Health Economics, University of York

Thomas Carlyle described economics as the 'dismal science' over one hundred years ago. Economics is concerned with how choices are made to allocate scarce resources amongst competing ends. The starting point for the economist is that resources are scarce, and that choices are unavoidable and should be made explicitly to foster efficiency and accountability.

In health care, the resource allocation issue becomes 'rationing': deciding who will be treated, who will be left untreated to live in pain and discomfort and, *in extremis,* who will be left to die. Such choices are unavoidable, but in health care are hedged round by the mystic of medicine and by individual and social reluctance to accept the one certainty in life—death. Ideally, scarce health care resources should be allocated to maximise improvements in 'health gain', and in the length and quality of life. A failure to behave efficiently (i.e. to improve health to the greatest extent at least cost) is unethical. A doctor who uses resources inefficiently deprives potential patients of care from which they could benefit. Why is the ideal of efficient practice so difficult to achieve?

Impediments to efficient resource allocation

There are many impediments to the achievement of efficiency in the allocation or rationing of health care resources. Three impediments are discussed here: ritual, ignorance and undue haste.

Ritual: the failure to evaluate common policy processes

Much of the discussion of National Health Service (NHS) policy is ritualised, with critical appraisal of its basis absent. A nice example of this is the annual process by which expenditure on the NHS is determined in Whitehall.

The demand for health care is growing more rapidly than society's willingness to fund it. Two important elements in demand growth are demography and technology change, both of which are dealt with superficially in most discussions of health care. For instance, in the annual UK expenditure round, the Department of Health 'bids' for increased funding for the elderly by multiplying the existing average expenditure on the elderly (65–74, 75–84, 85 years and over) by the increase in the number of elderly (0.5% in 1993–94). There is no evidence that the existing average expenditure is efficient, and little evidence about the cost-effectiveness of most of the services provided for the elderly. The Department of Health estimates, and the Treasury accepts, without any scientific basis, that technology change requires a 0.5% increase in real expenditure annually. The Department has 'played this game' for over a decade and made no serious attempt to validate it.

So, whilst the conventional wisdom is that the increasing numbers and dependency of the elderly and the rising tide of technological advance both necessitate real increases in funding, a precise knowledge base to inform the annual public expenditure 'cycle' is absent. The annual public expenditure round is a ritual in which policy assumptions are not evaluated, and the consequent discourse about NHS funding remains naive and limited. Thus, the Department of Health and the Treasury continue to practise Marxism!

> The secret of life is honesty and fair play. If you can fake that, you've made it.
>
> Groucho Marx

Ignorance: 'what works' in medicine?

However, the Department of Health and the Treasury are not the only Marxists in town! The members of the medical profession are also practised exponents of this process of faking (defined in the Oxford Dictionary as 'contriving out of poor material'). As patients, we all want to believe that what is to be done to us will remedy our ills and give us everlasting life. Unfortunately, the knowledge base to support these beliefs is absent.

Trial design. The design and implementation of clinical trials are often inadequate. A trial may be well designed in terms of patient entry criteria, statistical size and the measurement of a narrow range of clinical end-points. However, such trials may not demonstrate whether the experimental treatment is cost-effective in comparison to the control. Indeed, some clinicians continue to assert that this information is not relevant. For instance, some cancer trialists believe that trial design should use large numbers to identify whether length of patient life is increased.

Is this the only relevant issue for making a choice? An NHS purchaser may ask at what cost are additional life-years produced? What is the quality of life for those additional life-years? The trial of the prophylactic use of tamoxifen will produce evidence about increased survival for women with a high risk of breast cancer. It will not produce cost and quality-of-life data because it is planned to produce those data later. Timing is of the essence! Will policy makers be able to restrain the prophylactic use of tamoxifen until cost and quality of life data are produced if enhanced survival is demonstrated? Experience tells us that the benefit maximisers will not be restrained by the needs of science and the requirements of purchasers.

Variation on practice. The extent of variations in medical practice is impressive because of the way clinical science has been developed and applied, and how doctors are trained. This may be illustrated with regard to cancer:

1. There are significant variations in the cost of cancer treatments; for example, the cost of radiotherapy was found to vary from £9 to £37 per fraction (1988 UK£) by Goddard and Hutton.[1]
2. Perhaps three-quarters of chemotherapy and half of radiotherapy treatments aim to palliate not to cure. Yet only recently have trials begun to focus on the effects of these interventions in terms of quality of life. The review by Morris of quality-of-life studies in the head and neck area showed that the majority of studies were retrospective, descriptive, based on small samples, and narrowly focused on functional disability only.[2]
3. Priestman *et al.* reported large variations in radiotherapy treatment; for example, for a 65-year-old woman with metastatic breast cancer experiencing pain, the clinical respondents offered 1 to 15 fractions, with a median of 5.[3] For a 50-year-old man with inoperable cancer of the bronchus with distressing symptoms, the survey revealed a treatment range of 1 to 36 fractions, with a median of 10. Patients with very similar illness characteristics clearly receive very different treatments.

Absence of outcome measurement. Why is it that so little effort is deployed to remedy the variations in clinical practice? Is it because of the absence of outcome measurement? To demonstrate a therapy is efficient, it is necessary to measure outcome and enhancements in both the length and quality of life. Florence Nightingale adopted a definition of outcome stated in the 1844 Lunacy Act and used in psychiatric hospitals throughout the 19th century: dead, relieved and unrelieved.[4] She went on to argue:

> I am fain to sum up with an urgent appeal for adopting this or some uniform system of publishing the statistical records of hospitals. There is a growing conviction that in all hospitals, even in those which are best conducted, there is a great and unnecessary waste of life . . .
>
> In attempting to arrive at the truth, I have applied everywhere for information but in scarcely an instance have I been able to obtain hospital records fit for any purpose of comparison. If they could be obtained, they would enable us to decide many other questions besides the ones alluded to. They would show subscribers how their money was being spent, what amount of good was really being done with it, or whether the money was doing mischief rather than good.

No hospital anywhere today measures outcomes in the way advocated by Nightingale. Where limited outcomes are measured, they appear to have few demonstrable effects on practice; for example, have the variations in avoidable mortality identified in the Confidential Enquiry into Perioperative Deaths (CEPOD) been removed? If it is asserted that they have, where is the evidence?

Purchasers in the newly reformed NHS are required to measure the health needs of the local population and to identify cost-effective procedures to meet those needs. Unfortunately, the knowledge base to do this is absent. Fuchs agreed that 10% of health care expenditure worsened patients' health, 10% had no effect and 80% improved health.[5] He argued that the problem is no one knows which therapies lie in the 10% and 80% categories! Cochrane[6] and Black[7] have also argued that only a small portion (10%) of health care practices are proven rather than experimental. No one, not even doctors, knows 'what works' in health care.

Undue haste in 'operationalising' rationing

Purchasers need to know the value both of what is given up (the opportunity cost) and of what is gained (the welfare arising from improved health) when deciding to invest their limited budgets in any therapy. They are often tempted to make undue haste, confusing activity with work. In so doing, they adopt superficial 'quick fixes', rather than create an explicit framework for choice informed by an iterative and careful quest for new knowledge, which exploits existing knowledge and ensures the development of good quality research to create new knowledge. Purchasers facing difficult choices are striving for this knowledge worldwide. For example:

- In New Zealand, a government committee is seeking to identify the 'core' of health services which should be funded by the state. This core is to be the set of therapies which can be proven to be cost-effective.
- In the Netherlands, the government committee on choices in health care hopes to identify that core of medical services which can be proven to be cost-effective.[8]
- In Oregon, the Health Commission drew up a ranked list of 709 condition–treatment pairs, and decided to draw its budget line for Medicaid patients at item 587. This process, which is discussed by Strosberg *et al.*,[9] involved exploitation of the limited evaluative literature, an appeal to medical consensus, the measurement of public opinions and, at the end, subjective manipulation of rankings.
- The UK equivalent of this search for the Holy Grail is measurement of outcomes in terms of the quality-adjusted life month (QALM) or quality-adjusted life year (QALY) (Table 1). These are now available from the Department of Health with 700 categories in a variety of therapeutic groups.

All these mechanisms are crude; for example, what are the confidence intervals for QALYs, and has there been careful appraisal of the studies from which they are derived? Do rankings alter if such appraisal is carried out?

The difficulty with operationalising rationing is that neither the medical profession nor other groups have created a knowledge base to make choices. As a result, policy makers use crude methods to meet an urgent and unavoidable purchaser need. They do this in great haste, tending to identify an 'urgent' need, and using limited methods to meet these needs. Rationing or prioritisation is a process where haste will produce limited results. Such activity is an iterative process where both careful exploitation of existing knowledge and adding to knowledge by well planned research create insights useful to purchasers. Those who search for the 'quick fix' may impair policy making and set back the search for new knowledge.

Improving the knowledge base

The need to invest in the systematic economic evaluation of both the opportunity cost and the health status improvement to improve the knowledge base is as great as it is for decisions about how to invest limited budgets in a therapy. There are four types of

Table 1. The cost per quality-adjusted life year (QALY) of competing therapies: some tentative estimates.

	Cost/QALY (£, Aug. 1990)
Cholesterol testing and diet therapy (all adults aged 40–69)	200
Neurosurgical intervention for head injury	240
General practitioner advice to stop smoking	270
Neurosurgical intervention for subarachnoid haemorrhage	490
Antihypertensive therapy to prevent stroke (all adults aged 45–64)	940
Pacemaker implantation	1100
Hip replacement	1180
Valve replacement for aortic stenosis	1410
Cholesterol testing and treatment (all adults aged 40–69)	1480
CABG (LMVD, severe angina)	2090
Kidney transplantation	4710
Breast cancer screening	5780
Heart transplantation	7840
Cholesterol testing and treatment (incrementally) (all adults aged 25–39)	14,150
Home haemodialysis	17,260
CABG (1-vessel disease, moderate angina)	18,830
Hospital haemodialysis	21,970
Erythropoietin treatment for anaemia in dialysis patients (assuming 10% reduction in mortality)	54,380
Neurosurgical intervention for malignant intracranial tumours	107,780
Erythropoietin treatment for anaemia in dialysis patients (assuming no increase in survival)	126,290

Sources: References 10–15.
CABG   = coronary artery bypass graft
LMVD   = left main vessel disease

economic evaluation (Table 2). The *cost-minimisation* technique involves the detailed costing of the alternatives, and is dependent on the assumption that their outcomes are identical. Unfortunately, the assumption of identical outcome is often not valued. Piachaud and Weddell evaluated the alternative ways of treating varicose veins—surgery versus injection compression sclerotherapy.[16] Using the best available clinical data, they assumed that

Table 2. Types of economic evaluation (cost measurement in £).

| | Outcome measurement | |
	What measured	How valued
Cost-minimisation	Assumed identical	None
Cost-benefit analysis	All effects produced by the alternative	£
Cost-effectiveness analysis	Single common specific variable; achieved to varying extents	Common units (e.g. life years)
Cost-utility analysis	Effects of the competing therapies; achieved to differing levels	QALYs

QALY = quality-adjusted life year

the outcomes were identical, costed the alternatives, and concluded that the non-surgical intervention was best. Within five years, the clinical knowledge basis had shifted, and surgery was shown to have superior outcomes, thus invalidating the conclusion of Piachaud and Weddell.

Cost-benefit analysis is the preferred form of economic evaluation for economists. However, it requires the identification, measurement and valuation of all costs and benefits in financial terms. The measurement of the value of life and of distress and pain avoided is a complex area, in which there is now renewed interest and experimentation, but at present the use of such techniques is quite limited in health care.[17]

Cost-effectiveness analysis involves the costing of the alternatives and the measurement of effectiveness in some simple unitary measure. For instance, in a pioneering economic evaluation, Klarman *et al.* investigated the costs and effects of two interventions for patients with end-stage renal failure—transplantation and dialysis.[18] They concluded that transplantation was the cheaper way of producing additional years of life, and added that the quality of survival with this option also appeared to be superior.

Such results are useful to inform choices between different types of treatment for chronic renal failure. A problem with this approach is that the effectiveness measure for other illnesses may be different; for example, for hypertension treatment, it might be blood pressure measured in terms of millimetres of mercury.

Consequently, it is difficult to compare effectiveness measures in chronic renal failure with effectiveness in hypertension control. The technique of cost-effectiveness analysis is thus useful to identify preferred treatments in particular therapeutic categories, but of little use in identifying the best value for money across all therapeutic options.

To overcome this limitation, a fourth technique of economic evaluation, *cost-utility* analysis, has been devised. This approach involves the identification of the full social costs of the alternative interventions, and the measurement of their effects with an outcome indicator which not only identifies the value of the enhancements in the length and quality of life but also does so in a way that can be used across therapeutic categories. This outcome measure is the QALY or healthy year equivalent (HYE), both of which measure the effectiveness of therapies in terms of their capacity to enhance both the length and the quality of life.

There is controversy about the accuracy and validity of QALYs and HYEs (see ref. 17 for a review), which is indicative of the need to have an agreed set of criteria to judge the quality of economic evaluations. If the purchasers of health care and regulators in the health care industry require to know what is good value for money, what should they look for when designing economic evaluations and assessing the validity of published results? Eight questions need to be addressed when evaluating all economic evaluations, some of which are similar to those addressed in clinical trials:

1. Are the research question and the trial design clearly identified and feasible?
2. Are both the experimental and control (comparator) arms of the trial well described?
3. Are all relevant costs of different decision making groups (e.g. the patient, his/her carers, the hospital, the health care system) and society identified, quantified and valued?
4. Are all the relevant effects (outcomes measured in terms of enhancements in the length and quality of life) of the competing therapies identified, quantified and valued?
5. Is the sample appropriate and sufficient in size to ensure statistical power for costs and effects?
6. Are marginal (incremental) costs and effects identified?
7. Are costs and effects discounted appropriately (to take account of time preference)?
8. Are the results subjected to sensitivity analysis?

Cost measurement

Perhaps the two most important elements in this list concern cost
and outcome measurement. The identification, measurement and
valuation of all the relevant costs of the alternative treatments are
complex. The purpose of any such costing is to identify the value
to society of the resources forgone in providing the intervention.
These societal costs will include the costs to the health care system,
both primary and hospital, the costs of statutory community support, of care provided by charities and the private sector, and to
the patient and his carers.

The interest of some groups may be in a subset of these costs
(e.g. the costs to the hospital). However, if studies are carried out
on subsets of costs relevant to health care purchasers in different
compartments of the health care system, inefficient decision making may result. A new therapy may reduce the costs of hospital care
but shift patients and costs on to health care sectors. A policy that
reduces costs for the hospital may increase costs for primary care,
the patient and his carers. If a societal approach to costing is not
taken, the resource consequences of such cost shifting will be
missed by the economic evaluation.

It is essential that all relevant costs are identified. When evaluating an economic evaluation, a list of relevant costs is to be expected as is the inevitability that some of these costs may not be mea-
surable and valued. For instance, a carer's input into a treatment
process (e.g. an elderly spouse caring for his wife) can be identified and measured in terms of leisure hours given up, but its value
is more difficult to ascertain. One approach is to use the value of
an alternative input (e.g. nursing) which might have to be provided in the absence of the carer.

Outcome measurement

The identification, measurement and valuation of all relevant
outcomes is one of the most contentious elements in any economic evaluation. In principle, the evaluation of the survival
element in outcome measurement is simple. In practice, it is difficult because mortality data are rarely linked and, as a consequence, whilst inpatient survival data may be available, these are
not linked to survival after discharge into the community. These
problems, in principle at least, can be resolved by better data collection, but the difficulties involved in the measurement of the
quality of life are both practical and methodological. There are
two parts in the process of quality of life measurement: selection

of descriptors, and selection of valuation methods.

The purpose of descriptor selection is to identify those characteristics of social, physical and psychological well-being which the population regard as appropriate to measure the quality of life. Physical characteristics may include elements such as the ability to get out of bed unaided, wash and dress, eat unassisted, walk up and down stairs and walk down the street. Psychological well-being descriptors may include aspects of everyday life such as feeling happy and having energy. Social well-being descriptors may appraise the individuals.

The selection of a set of descriptors should not be arbitrary and decided unilaterally by the investigator. Careful measurement of social attitudes to alternative descriptors is necessary. Whatever set of descriptors is selected, various combinations of social, physical and psychological aspects of the quality of life are possible. How are these alternative combinations to be valued? The preferred valuation methods are the time trade off and standard gamble approaches, although there is no consensus as to which is the superior.[19]

There are many quality-of-life measures to choose from, most of them disease-specific, and the extent to which they are validated is incomplete.[20,21] The number of generic quality-of-life measures which can be used across diagnostic categories is small, for example, SF36 (Short Form 36),[22] the EuroQol,[23] the Nottingham Health Profile (NHP), the Quality of Well-Being (QWB), and the Sickness Impact Profile (SIP).[19] The validity of these generic measures is gradually being explored more extensively. Many pharmaceutical companies are using SF36, and the instrument has now been translated from American into Swedish, German, French and English. However, it contains some interesting assumptions, for example, that the weights of all descriptors are equal. The empirical basis for this assumption appears to be untested: do populations regard being able to get up and dress as equally important as being able to walk a block?[24] Also, there are different variants of SF36 in which the descriptors are the same but the algorithms used to compute values vary.

Another important aspect of outcome measurement is whether enhancements in the length and quality of life are of equal value to society if they accrue to patient groups of different ages. Is an additional year of good quality of life for a 75-year-old equal in value to the same gain for a 25-year-old? Many studies assume such gains are of equal value, regardless of the beneficiary's age, but available empirical evidence does not sustain this position. An explicit social debate about such weighting is appropriate.

These and other issues in quality of life measurement make the subject and the practice contentious. There is no 'gold standard' measure, and the best practice is to use a validated disease-specific measure alongside a generic measure. When evaluating economic evaluations, the reader should focus sharply on how outcomes were measured. If the eight questions listed above are used to inform the design of trials and to evaluate their results, economic evaluation will improve the knowledge base and gradually inform purchaser choices more fully.

Application of these techniques is an iterative process. Critical evaluation of studies will identify their weaknesses, which should stimulate the improvement of methods and new applied studies. Adequate models for economic evaluation exist, and it is not premature to invest in these substantially (rather than tentatively and inadequately as now) to inform choice making in the NHS.

Conclusions

Existing rationing methods in all health care systems are incoherent, implicit and indefensible. The medical profession has served its own and society's interests poorly by failing to evaluate how well its members spend £35 billion. It is not known 'what works' in health care, and the practice of medical practitioners varies substantially within hospitals, and between districts, regions and countries. Most medical practice appears to be experimental and urgently in need of evaluation in terms of its costs and benefits. The process of remedying these grave deficiencies requires doctors and all other researchers to follow carefully the dictum of Chairman Mao:

> Knowledge is a matter of science, and no dishonesty or conceit whatsoever is permissible. What is required is definitely the reverse: honesty and modesty.

Let us look forward to honesty and modesty in health services research in the 1990s.

References

1. Goddard M, Hutton J. What is the cost of radiotherapy? *European Journal of Radiology* 1991; **13**: 76–9.
2. Morris J. *The quality of life of head and neck cancer patients: a review of the literature. Discussion paper 72.* York: Centre for Health Economics, University of York, 1990.
3. Priestman TJ, Bullimore JA, Goddern TP, Deutsch GP. The Royal College of Radiologists Fractionation Study. *Clinical Oncology* 1989; **1**: 63–6.

4. Nightingale F. *Some notes on nursing.* London: Longmans Green, 1863.
5. Fuchs V. Rationing health care. *New England Journal of Medicine* 1984; **311**: 1572–3.
6. Cochrane AL. *Effectiveness and efficiency.* London: Nuffield Provincial Hospitals Trust, 1972.
7. Black AD. *An anthology of false antitheses. Rock Carling 1984 Fellowship.* London: Nuffield Provincial Hospitals Trust, 1986.
8. Government Committee on Choices in Health Care. *Choices in health care. Dunning Report.* Rijswijk, Netherlands: Ministry of Welfare, Health and Cultural Affairs, 1992.
9. Strosberg MA, Wiener JM, Baker R, Fein IA, eds. *Rationing America's health care: the Oregon plan and beyond.* Washington DC: Brookings Institute, 1992.
10. Department of Health and Social Security. *Breast cancer screening. Forrest Report.* London: HMSO, 1986.
11. Department of Health, Standing Medical Advisory Committee. *Blood cholesterol testing: the cost-effectiveness of opportunistic cholesterol testing.* London: Department of Health, 1990.
12. Leese B, Hutton J, Maynard A. *The costs and benefits of the use of erythropoietin in the treatment of anaemia arising from chronic renal failure.* York: Centre for Health Economics, University of York. Occasional paper, 1990.
13. Pickard JD, Bailey S, Sanderson H, Rees M, Garfield JS. Steps towards cost-benefit analysis of regional neurosurgical care. *British Medical Journal* 1990; **301**: 629–35.
14. Teeling Smith G. The economics of hypertension and stroke. *American Heart Journal* 1990; **119** (Suppl): 725–8.
15. Williams A. Economics of coronary artery bypass grafting. *British Medical Journal* 1985; **249**: 326–9.
16. Piachaud D, Weddell JM. The economics of treating varicose veins. *International Journal of Epidemiology* 1972; **1**: 287–94.
17. Hutton J. Cost-benefit analysis of health care expenditure decision making. *Health Economics* 1992; **1**: 213–6.
18. Klarman HE, Francis JO'S, Rosenthal GD. Cost effectiveness analysis applied to the treatment of chronic renal failure. *Medical Care* 1968; **6**: 48–54.
19. Kind P. *The design and construction of quality of life measures. Discussion paper 43.* York: Centre for Health Economics, University of York, 1988.
20. Fallowfield L. *The quality of life: the missing measurement in health care.* London: Souvenir Press, 1990.
21. Spilker B, Molinek FR, Johnston KA, Simpson RL, Tilson HH. Quality of life bibliography and indexes. *Medical Care* 1990; **28** (12) (Suppl): 1–77.
22. Stewart AL, Ware JE, eds. *Measuring functioning and well-being: the medical outcomes study approach.* Durham, NC: Duke University Press, 1992.
23. EuroQol Group. EuroQol—a new facility for the measurement of health related quality of life. *Health Policy* 1990; **16**: 199–208.
24. Williams A. Review article on: Measuring functioning and well-being: the medical outcomes study approach, Stewart AL, Ware JE, eds. *Health Economics* 1992; **4**: 255–8.

2 | The Oregon experience

E Paul Kirk
*Chairman and Professor, Department of Obstetrics and Gynecology,
Oregon Health Sciences University, Portland, Oregon, USA
Chairman, Oregon Health Services Commission 1992–93*

In discussing the Oregon experience in the context of the
rationing of health care in medicine, it is necessary (first) to make
some preliminary comments about the American health care system and to try to explain why the Oregon Plan was suggested. It is
not possible to present a full and detailed discussion of the
methodology, but I will try to give sufficient detail to understand
the political dilemma currently faced by the plan's architects.
Finally, I will attempt some predictions as to what its future might
be in the light of the recent presidential election.

Health care in the USA

The Oregon Plan is one of many that have been presented over
the last couple of years as ways not necessarily of solving the multi-
faceted health care crisis in the USA but as a mechanism for dealing with a local problem—one that is admittedly illustrative of a
particular defect in the national system. This defect is access to
care or, more properly, timely access to care. In the USA, care is
provided, but for many access to it is difficult and often postponed.
Access may be through the emergency services at a time of crisis,
rather than through a primary care provider when the opportunity
for earlier intervention might have prevented a later, more critical
problem. The essential reason why so many people have difficulty
with access is not lack of facilities or lack of providers, but an
inability to pay for the service either directly by paying the fee-for-
service, or indirectly through one of the many different forms of
insurance emerging from the traditional indemnity insurance of
Blue Cross and Blue Shield to the insurer/providers of the health
maintenance organisations such as Kaiser.

The evolution of the American system has been well described by Paul Starr in his book, *The social transformation of American Medicine,*[1] and by David Rothman in *Strangers at the bedside.*[2] Starr describes the development of a massive health care industry, while Rothman discusses the modification of the doctor–patient relationship by a 'bewildering number of parties and procedures participating in medical decision making'. Starr describes the transition in the first half of the century from out-of-pocket payment of fees for services where options were limited and costs relatively low, through the establishment of insurers for hospital and provider payments, and the assumptions of the cost of the insurance by employers during World War II. In the 1960s, the federal government stepped in to provide coverage for the elderly through Medicare, and to the poor through Medicaid. The states have been allowed wide discretion as to how they define 'poor', so there are wide variances in eligibility rules from state to state. The federal government has not, however, allowed discretion as to the services covered, 'mandating' that the states provide the service that it insists upon rather than those the states select.

Although the system evolved in the hope that all citizens would be covered either by their work-based insurance or by government programmes, including the Veterans' Administration and the Indian Health Service as well as Medicare and Medicaid, the reality has been far from the dream. For a while, the system worked because most people were covered, the industry turned a profit, and costs could be shifted from the insured to pay for the charity care of those who were falling through the cracks in the existing system. This 'charity care' suited the complex American personality: a fierce belief in individualism, competition, the marketplace, 'can-doism', and profit but, at the same time, the recognition that some of the profit should be directed to caring for the needy. This informal system began to disintegrate as costs escalated. The incentive of fee-for-service encouraged the provision of as many services as possible; the separation of the patient from the bill by the third-party insurance companies also encouraged consumption, the technological explosion raised expectations and provided more opportunities and, as the industry responded, its bureaucracy expanded with it. As costs increased, employers were less able to provide work-based insurance, and a new class of patients appeared—the 'working uninsured'—families who were poor, but not so poor that they qualified for Medicaid, and whose breadwinners were working, but not for employers who were willing or able to provide them with the euphemistically termed 'fringe' benefits of health insurance.

Background to the Oregon Plan

For many, then, one part of the American dream—immediate access to superb health care of individual choice—became the reality of the fear of family illness with no insurance and with care beyond their reach. One such family facing this reality in 1987 was Coby Howard's. Eight-year-old Coby had leukemia, and his single mother was a Medicaid recipient. A request was made to Oregon's legislative emergency board for Coby to go out of state for a bone marrow transplant. The request was denied, and Coby died. The $180,000 that could have been spent on his transplant was allocated to prenatal care. The decision, the circumstances in which it was made, and the credentials and competency of the decision makers were widely criticised. To their credit, the state legislature did not let the matter rest and, under the leadership of John Kitzhaber, the Oregon Plan was developed. The principles on which it was founded are shown in Table 1.

Three bills were introduced to the state legislature: one to focus on the Medicaid population (Senate Bill 27), another to focus on the working uninsured by the establishment of a state insurance pool to which employers would have to contribute if they were not providing insurance, and the third to provide coverage for individuals with chronic illness (persons who often had difficulty in obtaining insurance because of their pre-existing conditions). The intentions of the basic Health Care Act are outlined in Table 2.

The current Medicaid system is cumbersome, inconsistent and insensitive. As already stated, the states have the discretion of defining their own eligibility rules. Oregon currently defines eligibility to 48% of the federal poverty level ($460/month for a family of three). Coverage is provided for children aged 7–18 in single-parent households or in two-parent households where certain financial criteria are met. The Oregon Plan, and the essence of its

Table 1. Oregon Plan principles (John Kitzhaber MD, 1989).

1. All citizens should have access to universal health care.
2. Process to determine basic care.
3. Process based on public debate of criteria.
4. Process should seek consensus of social values.
5. Process should consider good of society as a whole.
6. Eligibility will be faced on financial need.
7. Mechanisms to establish accountability for resource allocation and consequences.

Table 2. Intentions: Oregon basic Health Care Act (Senate Bill 27).

- Fixes income level to qualify at 100% of federal poverty level.
- Providers reimbursed at cost or higher.
- Encourages 'managed health care'.
- Established Health Services Commission to develop a prioritised list of health services.
- Established a methodology to adjust benefit package based on the amount of money available.

controversy, was to extend the population covered to include older children and adults, and to bring eligibility up to 100% of the federal poverty level. In order to do this, a Health Services Commission was appointed by the Governor, consisting of five physicians, a medical social worker, a public health nurse, and four consumers. The Commission was given a seductively simple task:

> to report to the Governor a list of health services ranked by priority from the most important to the least important representing the comparative benefits of each service to the entire population to be served.

Once the list was constructed, it was to be submitted to actuarial analysis so that the Oregon legislature would have to make a decision where to 'draw the line'. Services above the line would be covered; those below the line would not. By placing more money into the programme, more services would be covered; by reducing the funding, fewer sevices would be available.

Public reactions to the Oregon Plan

From the outset, the plan provoked many and varied reactions. With some exceptions, there was fairly widespread local support, but it was soon evident that there were strong and vocal opponents outside the state. These voices were important because, although the plan was a local initiative to local access problems, it was necessary to have approval from the federal government so that the 'mandated services' could be waived. The federal government pays two out of every three dollars of Medicaid costs, so the state needed federal support in cash as well as in principle, and was in no position to 'go it alone' without federal permission.

Those in favour of the plan recognised that it was a genuine attempt to improve access, honest in that it recognised the inevitable clash between expectations and resources, and acknowledged the government's responsibility to spend the taxpayers' money as efficiently and effectively as possible. Supporters also recognised the broad coalition of different interest groups which had come together to help move the bill through the Oregon legislature. There was particularly enthusiastic support for that part of the legislation that required the Commission to incorporate the 'community's values' into its decision making process. Rather quaintly, a federal government report opined that the plan 'was not irrational'.

The critics raised a number of objections and protests. Activists for national health care reform objected to the incremental approach represented by the Oregon Plan and feared that it might distract from other more important proposals. In particular, some opponents objected that the plan was not cost-cutting. Indeed, the intention to reimburse 'at cost' was designed to increase access by limiting the cost shift. Some critics said that to rank services was either impossible or unethical, although the 'ethical' justification for the current system was rarely explained in counter argument. Ranking of services also caused anxiety and concern because it inevitably raised questions about the 'importance' of service at both ends of life—to the extremely premature infant and to the terminally ill adult. These concerns, and objections arising from them, were extended by some to include opposition to the inclusion on the list of abortion and contraception services. Other people, particularly those who had fought for the current mandates for women and children, feared the loss of some important services and resisted the waivers.

Methodology

Against this background, the Commission developed a methodology.[3] A health service was defined generally as an 'intervention expected to maintain and/or to restore health or well-being', and specifically as a treatment taken from the Physicians Current Procedural Terminology (CPT-4). Each procedure with its CPT code was linked with the diagnosis that it treated, forming a diagnosis–treatment pair. Where appropriate, more than one diagnosis and more than one treatment or pair were grouped together to form a 'line' on the list, which eventually totalled 708 lines.

The legislation that created the Health Services Commission required that:

> the Commission shall actively solicit public involvement in a community meeting process to reach a consensus on the values to be used to guide health resource allocation decisions.

· This public involvement was obtained in a number of ways:

- 12 public meetings were held at various locations around the state, and the general public was offered the opportunity of testifying on health care issues in general, but on the basic health care plan in particular;
- a telephone survey was conducted in which 1,001 respondents were asked to place a numerical value (0 = death to 100 = perfect health) on a list of symptoms and functional impairments, thereby rating the severity of the condition and establishing a modification of the Quality of Well-Being Scale described by Kaplan;[4]
- Oregon Health Decisions, a coalition representing a variety of organisations and individuals interested in society's input into health care reform, held 47 community meetings and, in their report to the Commission, provided a 'perspective' describing the values most frequently discussed by the 1,000 or more citizens who attended their meetings.

The list of values, and the frequency with which they were discussed, is given in Table 3.

Table 3. The values placed upon health care issues, and the frequency with which they were discussed, at public meetings in Oregon.

Value	Frequency
Prevention	Very high
Quality of life	Very high
Cost-effectiveness	High
Ability to function	Moderately high
Equity	Moderately high
Effectiveness of treatment	Medium high
Benefits many	Medium
Mental health and chemical dependency	Medium
Personal choice	Medium
Community compassion	Medium low
Impact on society	Medium low
Length of life	Medium low
Personal responsibility	Medium low

Very high	= all community meetings
High	= more than 75%
Moderately high	= 75%
Medium high	= more than 50%
Medium	= 50%
Medium low	= less than 50%

The lines (diagnosis–treatment pairs or groups) were placed in one of 17 categories which were then ranked (Table 4). To begin the category ranking process, each commissioner gave a relative weight from zero to 100 to the attributes of:

- value to society;
- value to an individual at risk of needing the service; and
- essential to a basic health care package.

These scores were used in a modified Delphi technique to produce the category rankings.

The help of medical experts was sought in establishing the net benefit and cost-benefit ratios for each diagnosis–treatment pair. Experts gave outcome probability data for mortality, return to former health state and morbidity. Up to three scenarios were chosen and described for each pair in addition to death and return to former health state. Using the weights obtained from the telephone survey for symptoms and functional impairment, a net benefit ratio was calculated as follows:

$$\text{Net benefit} = \frac{\text{With treatment}}{\text{Outcome} \times \text{Probability}} - \frac{\text{Without treatment}}{\text{Outcome} \times \text{Probability}}$$

The initial intention of calculating the cost-benefit ratio was abandoned because of the lack of reliable data regarding cost. Charge data were available but they were not used.

The diagnosis–treatment pairs and groups were ranked within their categories according to the calculated net benefit. This process resulted in a draft list. The commissioners used a 'reasonableness' test when they adjusted the objectively ranked health services. The health impact, cost of medical treatment, incidence of condition, effectiveness of treatment, social costs, and cost of non-treatment were used to determine a new ranking. The commissioners also observed that it was not reasonable—logically or economically—to rank preventable or readily treatable conditions in relatively unfavourable positions; in other words, where severe or exacerbated conditions were ranked in a relatively favourable position compared to prevention of disease, disability or exacerbation, their positions were reversed. When the list was finalised, it was sent to the actuaries for costing so that the Oregon legislature could allocate funds and determine the level at which the line was to be drawn.

Basic care

In presenting the list to the Governor, the Commission had

Table 4. Essential components of basic health care.

1. Acute fatal conditions for which treatment prevents death and provides full recovery: e.g. repair of deep open wound of the neck, appendectomy, and medical therapy for myocarditis.
2. Maternity care, including disorders of the newborn: e.g. obstetric care, medical therapy both for drug reactions and intoxications specific to newborns, and for low birthweight babies.
3. Acute fatal conditions for which treatment prevents death, but for which recovery is limited: e.g. surgical treatment for head injury with prolonged loss of consciousness, medical therapy for acute bacterial meningitis, and reduction of open fracture of a joint.
4. Preventive care for children: e.g. immunisations, medical therapy for streptococcal sore throat and scarlet fever, and screening for specific problems such as vision and hearing problems, or anaemia.
5. Chronic conditions that are fatal, and for which treatment improves lifespan and quality of life: e.g. medical therapy for type-1 diabetes mellitus, medical and surgical treatment for treatable cancer of the uterus, and medical therapy for asthma.
6. Reproductive services: e.g. contraceptive management, vasectomy, and tubal ligation.
7. Comfort care: e.g. palliative therapy for conditions in which death is imminent.
8. Preventive dental care for adults and children: e.g. cleaning and fluoride treatments.
9. Preventive care of proven efficacy for adults: e.g. mammograms, blood pressure screening, medical therapy, and chemoprophylaxis for primary tuberculosis.
10. Acute non-fatal conditions for which treatment is likely to bring a return to previous health: e.g. medical therapy for acute thyroiditis and for vaginitis, and restorative dental service for caries.
11. Chronic non-fatal conditions for which a one-time treatment improves the quality of life: e.g. hip replacement, laser surgery for diabetic retinopathy, and medical therapy for rheumatic fever.
12. Acute non-fatal conditions for which treatment is unable fully to restore previous health: e.g. arthroscopic repair of internal derangement of the knee, and repair of corneal laceration.
13. Chronic non-fatal conditions for which repetitive treatment improves the quality of life: e.g. medical therapy for chronic sinusitis, migraine headaches, and psoriasis.
14. Acute conditions that are non-fatal and self-limited, for which treatment expedites recovery: e.g. medical therapy for diaper rash, acute conjunctivitis, and pharyngitis.
15. Infertility services: e.g. medical therapy for anovulation, microsurgery for tubal disease, and *in vitro* fertilisation.
16. Preventive services of unproven benefit for adults: e.g. dipstick urinalysis for haematuria in adults less than 60 years of age, sigmoidoscopy for persons less than 40 years of age, and screening on non-pregnant adults for type-1 diabetes mellitus.
17. Fatal or non-fatal conditions for which treatment provides minimal or no improvement in quality of life: e.g. fingertip avulsion repair that does not include fingernail, medical therapy for gallstones without cholecystitis, and for viral warts.

struggled with the perceived need, often expressed at the public meetings, to define the precise content of basic health care. The Commission had no difficulty in thoroughly supporting the principle of making basic health services available to all or in establishing a definition of basic health care—that level of services below which no one should fall. At a philosophical level, the basic health care issue was fairly straightforward but, at a practical level, the Commission found it much more difficult to describe the content of that basic care, given both the format of the list and the uncertainty of the state's ability to fund any particular level. The resolution was to urge coverage for all services in categories considered essential and most of those in the categories considered very important. The Commission recognised that a definition of basic health care along these lines established a working model of basic care from society's viewpoint, but one that could not cover every individual contingency.

In July 1991, the legislature voted to increase its Medicaid funding by $28 million (a 15% increase), drawing the line at number 578 of the 708, with the result that 98% of the items in the essential category and 82% in the very important category were covered, but only 7% of the items in the categories considered important to the individual. By summer 1991, therefore, Oregon was ready to apply to the federal government for permission to start the programme, and the Governor wrote to the Secretary of the Department of Health and Human Services requesting waivers from the Medicaid mandates.

Political context

As Oregon waited, the presidential election campaign (a seemingly interminable process) commenced, and the debate about health care reform took centre stage. The Oregon Plan was used either to illustrate the virtues of acknowledging the inevitability of rationing and the importance of following an explicit process in establishing priorities, or to demonstrate the dangers of a public process which permitted a formal system for denying care—a position that usually chose to ignore the need to explain the current haphazard systems of implicit rationing.

The federal government took a year to decide whether to allow the experiment. In August 1992, the application was denied 'at least until a number of legal issues which relate primarily to the Americans with Disabilities Act are resolved'. In particular, the legal opinion found the use of the telephone survey discriminatory because it asked respondents to rate certain states of life on a scale of 0–100, with 100 representing perfect health.

The Health Services Commission members were aware of some of the potential abuse of quality-adjusted life years and similar indices as measures of outcomes, and had used these measures only as a device to measure the effectiveness of care, so they objected to the legal opinion that their process was discriminatory. Nevertheless, the list was redeveloped by means of a methodology which utilised only the avoidance of death and 'improvement' as indices (without attempting to quantify or qualify the health state itself or the type of improvement). The revised list contains 688 rather than 708 lines, there are a number of changes of sequence in the higher ranked diagnosis–treatment pairs and, with the new line being drawn at 587, 31 diagnosis–treatment pairs have gained coverage and 32 lost it.

The future

At this stage, it seems unlikely that the Oregon Plan will be implemented. Even though the methodology has been revised, so that it is presumably no longer in violation of the Americans with Disabilities Act, there is no incentive for the departing administration to grant the waivers. The new administration sees more comprehensive health care as part of its mandate, so the Oregon proposal has lost its significance.

Has it all been worthwhile? The experience has taken what to Americans is a dirty word—rationing—out of the closet and demonstrated that it is possible both to conduct a public discussion about values and to utilise the conclusion of those discussions. It has demonstrated that it will be difficult to measure effectiveness of care in anything other than the crudest of terms for fear of the accusation of discrimination. The plan's admittedly weak methodology has demonstrated the limitations of the available information about health care outcomes and lists. Even though the Oregon proposal may not be *the answer*, the question it asks—'What are our priorities and how do we order them?'—will have to be answered some time in the future. The proponents of the Oregon Plan would argue that sooner would be better than later.

Added in proof. The federal government finally granted the Medicaid waivers on 19 March 1993, conditional upon some further, minor modifications of the methodology used to formulate the list.

References

1. Starr P. *The social transformation of American medicine.* New York: Basic Books (Harper Collins), 1982.
2. Rothman D. *Strangers at the bedside.* New York: Basic Books (Harper Collins), 1991.
3. Oregon Health Services Commission. *Prioritization of health services: a report to the governor and legislature.* Portland, Oregon: Oregon Health Services Commission, 1989.
4. Kaplan RM, Anderson JP. General health policy manual: update and applications. *Health Services Research* 1988; **23:** 203–35.

3 | Decision making and the National Health Service: making choices in the real world—a philosophical approach

Kenneth C Calman
Chief Medical Officer, Department of Health

It has always been necessary to make decisions about the use of resources in the National Health Service (NHS). Making choices is not new, and neither therefore are the issues which lie behind the current debate about how the best and most efficient use can be made of the resources we have. The issues are essentially ethical or moral, and reflect the fact that if resources are finite, and demand exceeds what is available, decisions will be made, whether consciously or unconsciously, which will allow some people to be treated and others not. Until recently, such decisions were generally made by doctors, who worked within available resources and made individual decisions about patient care. This inevitably resulted in anomalies, in that some doctors were more successful than others in generating resources. In addition, skills and facilities varied from place to place, so rationing and variation in resources were geographically determined. The introduction of the NHS reforms has made these differences visible, and the debate has intensified as a result.

The role of ethics in health care is, first, to clarify thinking about the topic, secondly, to assist in the analysis of the issues involved and to dissect the problem and, finally, to provide the individual or organisation with a rational way in which to defend a particular course of action, based on the first two parts of the role. Different views may still result from the same analysis, so the key issue is the basic value base held by the individual or organisation. Thus, beliefs or values on social justice, personal responsibility for actions or public service will influence conclusions. For this reason, differences are likely to remain, but the issues will be clearer. This chapter sets out some of the areas to be considered, and provides a framework for making decisions. It inevitably reflects a personal view, though this has been minimised as far as possible. It should, however, provide a document for discussion.

The basic issues

Perhaps the first issue to discuss is the term 'resource'. This may be narrowly interpreted in terms of funding, or more widely in terms of skills, facilities or professional time available. This wider definition opens up other questions about individual professional responsibility in keeping up to date and providing a high quality service. It also raises the question as to how much resource in financial terms is available for the health service, and how and by whom that fundamental decision is made. Comparisons, crude though they may be, between different countries, suggest that there are different values. How consciously are these big decisions made? Are they based on rational arguments? Have we got it right, and others got it wrong? Comparisons are also interesting in relation to the technology available. Should liver and small bowel transplantation be available in this country because it is available in the USA? How many computerised tomography scanners should we have? Are there logical ways of deciding? What *can* the public expect, and what *do* they expect from the health service? How are these expectations raised, and what public debate should go on to inform them? Do we need some form of 'Oregon' debate in this country? Without trying to answer some of these questions, rationing will not be rational and it will become increasingly difficult to justify decisions.

The ethical framework

A number of basic ethical or moral principles can be set out. However, it will become clear that these can be, and sometimes are, conflicting. At the end of the day, the decision made on a particular issue will always be a matter of judgement. Consideration of the following principles should assist in maximising the clarity of the final decision and reduce uncertainty.

Justice

Justice is a basic value, and can relate to social factors, human rights and other issues. It is about fairness in dealing with all people equally. In health terms, it is about ensuring that there is equal access to health care, and that what is provided is of equal benefit.

Beneficence

Beneficence is about 'doing good', and is fundamental in any caring society. It is a positive value which ensures that all citizens have a place in society. But it is more than this: it expresses a feeling that society should help others, even those who may have 'opted out' or whose personal behaviour may be undesirable.

Non-maleficence

The principle of non-maleficence is about not doing harm to an individual or community. It is at its most obvious in relation to treatment programmes where a particular therapy may be harmful, but it is also relevant to, and may conflict with, beneficence. Research programmes or the introduction of a new procedure have both predictable and unpredictable effects. Society would not normally consciously introduce a technology which would harm an individual without full information being available.

Utility

Utility is simply stated as providing the greatest good for the greatest number. Applying this principle in relation to resource allocation with finite resources implies that their use should ensure that the greatest benefit results. Thus, some sections of the population may not be treated or investigated. There is conflict here with the principles of justice and beneficence. It may, however, be the key principle in relation to making choices.

Autonomy

The final principle, autonomy, emphasises the freedom and rights of the individual. For the individual human being, this principle implies that every person is entitled to all available resources. It is perhaps the value most often evoked when an individual requests or demands treatment. It is often in direct conflict with utility, and it is this more than anything which crystallises the dilemmas of resource allocation: how to support the autonomy and the rights of an individual when resource limitation means that the principles of utility and justice are also fundamental.

The way ahead

In trying to find a way through the issues which may, and do, arise the following framework is suggested based on three principles. The first is a graded series of health care interventions, based on the principles of justice and utility. The second is based on a determination of outcome and the benefit of the proposed intervention. Indeed, if there was certainty about the outcomes, decisions would be relatively easy. It is the *un*certainty which makes decisions difficult. Thus, the real need is for better outcome measures, and the conflicts are likely to continue until they are available. The third principle is to convert this information into economic terms, to be used for resource allocation. This is not considered further in this paper.

The following framework is therefore put forward as part of the debate and as a way of developing a comprehensive health service. Its purpose is to identify a series of categories related to health care in order to clarify both those issues about which it is relatively easy to make decisions and also others where decisions will remain difficult. Its purpose is therefore to reduce, but not eliminate, uncertainty, recognising that there may be variations in interpretation and resource allocation.

The framework

A caring society

All individuals in society have a right to be cared for. This does not mean that all individuals have a right to treatment or to institutional care, but that in any caring society arrangements are made to ensure that those in need are provided with comfort and support. It is the principle (beneficence) which is important, the public recognition that to be cared for when required will be a basic value of society. Traditionally, this was within the family, and there was a recognition that one or more members would be available to look after children, the disabled, the elderly and the sick.

Public health matters

All individuals have a right to have clean and safe water, air and food, secure housing and access to all evaluated and effective preventive and screening procedures. These public health issues underpin the process of maintaining good health and preventing illness. Immunisation is perhaps the clearest example of such an intervention. As ill health can be related to environmental issues interpreted in this broad way, it is relevant to ensure that the intervention is provided when it results in a benefit to health. The problem arises when an intervention, although beneficial, is relevant only to a small group of the population, and is therefore expensive. An example of this would be the screening of blood for a very rare infection. This would be beneficial, but very expensive and of value to a very small number of people, and it would divert resources from other areas—the principle of utility. It may be necessary to consider some rules, publicly debated, for dealing with such issues.

A primary care service

A primary care service is also a fundamental part of a comprehensive service. It would include child health, maternity services, care of the elderly and community care, provide individuals and families with a front-line service to deal with the majority of illnesses, and ensure that health promotional efforts are delivered. This country is fortunate in having perhaps the best developed primary care service in the world.

Accident and emergency services

The accident and emergency services would provide a trauma service, and facilities for dealing with emergency problems and acute life-saving issues such as heart attacks. In general, such services are not as well developed as they might be and are patchy around the country. Yet they should be seen as a basic part of providing a comprehensive health service.

Hospital-based services of proven value

The area where there is most to gain by a proper assessment of outcome and from savings in the elimination of ineffective procedures is the hospital-based services. Many investigations and treatments currently available are likely to be of unproven value. Fortunately, in this country at present there is no financial advantage to an individual doctor in carrying out a procedure, so decisions are made on clinical grounds alone. However, there is a major need to review all clinical practice and to ensure that only effective procedures are used The objective of such a review is certainly not to inhibit new developments or to prevent unproven treatments being used, but to recognise that such assessment needs to be done and to fund it accordingly. There is a strong argument for clinical guidelines in this area and for outcome measures to be used routinely—hence the importance of the Central Health Monitoring Unit, the Outcomes Unit, the initiatives on clinical audit, and the establishment of a Clinical Outcomes Group.

Expensive or special services planned on a national basis

Many services now available require special expertise, equipment or support services. Examples are expensive imaging techniques, some diagnostic methods, cardiac services, neonatal intensive care and many others. Effective outcomes rely on expertise and a sufficient throughput of patients to maintain the standards. It will be inefficient, therefore, to allow such services to develop on an unplanned basis. The educational implications of such decisions need to be considered.

New procedures to be evaluated on a research basis

In any comprehensive and developing health service, research and development are essential. It needs, however, to progress on a planned basis, and the Research and Development Division of the Department of Health has the framework in place to deliver this. It must be part of the culture to evaluate any service provided, and continually to improve the care provided. For professional staff, this is a central part of their work, and links to outcome measurement and clinical audit.

Conclusions

A number of general conclusions may be drawn from this brief discussion, based on a general acceptance of the framework presented. It should be stressed again that this chapter is not meant to be prescriptive, but rather to narrow the areas of uncertainty. The conclusions are based on the two principles outlined earlier: categorisation of issues, and assessment of outcomes.

1. There should be general agreement that society has a role in the care of its citizens, and that provision should be made for this through a range of mechanisms.
2. There is a need to be clear about which public health measures should be offered, based on an assessment of effectiveness. Such measures include environmental issues, immunisation, safety aspects and screening. Health promotional activities should be evaluated in the same way as other topics.
3. The primary care infrastructure should be developed and supported. It is the basis for the provision of health care. Much greater use could be made of the information available from the primary care team in the planning of health care. It is essential that in primary care, as in hospital-based medicine, procedures of known value are used. Classification of treatment procedures would be an important part of this.

4. Accident and emergency services are known to vary in efficiency
    and effectiveness. More needs to be done to define what is avail-
    able, what is of value, and how it should be provided. This would
    reduce both mortality and disability.

5. Within the hospital sector, it is essential to classify investiga-
    tions and treatments according to whether or not they are of
    value. It is realised that this is a major task, and that there will
    be grey areas. That, however, is not an excuse. Already a great
    deal of work has been done, and with the tools currently avail-
    able can be taken much further—because more needs to be
    done. If greater effectiveness is to be achieved within the
    health service, an assessment of the outcome and value of a
    procedure or treatment is at the heart of the process.

6. There will always be expensive or special procedures for which
    particular resources, including skills and facilities, are re-
    quired. For this reason, it remains necessary to plan these
    nationally to ensure their best use. Fragmentation of these
    resources will be wasteful nationally, and is one argument for a
    'managed market'.

7. There needs to be a more clearly defined list of procedures of a
    research nature, which are thus in the process of evaluation, and
    of those which are within established practice. There is a clear
    public dimension to this, in that the public need to be aware of
    what is 'available' within the NHS, and what will be available
    only to a limited number as the procedure is developed.

    There are also professional and managerial dimensions to
    this. Doctors and others should be encouraged to try new tech-
    niques and to modify existing ones, in an attempt to improve
    care, but this process has to be managed in order to gain the
    maximum amount of information. Managers must be able to
    encourage initiative and to realise that one of their roles is the
    improvement of health care. In so doing, they will recognise
    that this has a cost.

8. Much of the discussion has been about how doctors and other
    professional staff perform. There is therefore an important
    educational dimension to making decisions and using
    resources. Discussions are already underway with the profes-
    sions on many of these matters, and they will continue.

9. In all the above there is an important public dimension. Some
    of the difficult concepts described in this chapter should be
    publicly debated in some way. In general, it would be best to do
    this in broad terms, rather than in relation to a specific, and
    almost certainly an emotive, issue.

Envoi

The key to resource allocation is based on an assessment of effectiveness and outcomes of intervention. This applies to intervention in primary and secondary care, public health and managerial initiatives. A further issue, not developed in this paper, is the translation of knowledge of effectiveness into economic terms. This second stage in the process is crucial if resource allocation is to be rationally based.

4 | Rationing in practice: acute medicine

Michael Tunbridge
Consultant Physician, Newcastle General Hospital,
Newcastle upon Tyne

One of the hallmarks of the National Health Service (NHS) has been its ability and willingness to cope with emergencies of any type, at any time of day or night. Most areas of this country are very fortunate in having a primary health care system unmatched by other countries. It is likely to be the family doctor who deals first with many of the emergencies and will selectively refer those patients who are thought to be in need of hospital treatment. The best place for such a patient to be received is the district general hospital (DGH), which is equipped with staff and facilities to provide appropriate care. It is the not unreasonable expectation of the public, whichever member of their family falls ill, with whatever condition, that the hospital service will respond, whether the patient is sent there by the family doctor or is self-referred to the accident and emergency (A&E) department. It is a further expectation both of the public and of the profession that patients who need hospital care will be admitted. Failure to provide such care would properly be a matter of censure by the public, the profession and politicians alike. Whilst there may be no intention to ration care of the acutely ill patient, nevertheless in practice there are constraints which have this effect.

This discussion will be confined to the medical rather than to the surgical aspects of acute emergencies because medicine does not fit the neat surgical models used as a basis for much of the present NHS reforms.

Definition of acute general (internal) medicine

It would be as well to try to define acute general (internal) medicine (acute G(I)M) before proceeding further. Outside the UK, it has been defined by the formula $1-\sigma_n$, where σ stands for each subspecialty of medicine, e.g. cardiology, neurology, etc., and general medicine is what is left—mainly connective tissue diseases.

33

This is far removed from the practice of acute G(I)M in the UK, where it may be defined as the sum of all the acute aspects of the specialties of medicine minus E, the elective work. As E is almost non-existent in acute G(I)M, E approximates to zero. Thus, acute general medicine may be summarised by the formula $\Sigma\sigma_n$.

The acute medical service in any hospital is expected to deal with any problems that arise in patients outwith the narrow boundaries defined by other disciplines. A typical emergency intake would include patients with heart attack, respiratory failure, gastrointestinal haemorrhage, metabolic disturbances, infections, stroke and often combinations of these conditions in one patient. It will also include the worrying non-specific condition known as 'off-legs', which may hide an enormous variety of sinister as well as simple underlying problems, particularly in the elderly. Acute medicine is not the glamorous 'high tech' aspect of health care but it is the sharp end.

Problems with acute general medicine

Demand

The major difficulty with acute medicine is that it is demand-led. Emergency admissions are dictated by the needs of the acutely ill patient, whether referred by the general practitioner (GP) or self-referred. There are also patients already in the hospital in other departments who develop complications which need the expertise of a physician.

Geographical constraints

Certain constraints on the availability of the acute medical service have always existed. Geography may in part determine whether someone, for example, in the remoter parts of Scotland, is best managed at home rather than being sent a long distance by road or even by air. Most of the population however lives within easier reach of a DGH.

Ambulance service

The ambulance service, applying its own rules, is required to deliver patients to the nearest hospital providing emergency services, regardless of whether or not the medical beds in that hospital are full.

Nursing staff

There are also constraints imposed by the lack of availability of nursing staff. It is commonplace to have only two nurses on duty on a medical ward at night. In an acute medical receiving ward, the heavy demands on the nursing staff required by acutely ill, often elderly, patients require a higher nurse-to-patient ratio than on other less acute wards, even if they do not reach the nurse-to-patient ratios required in an intensive care unit. Lack of availability of nurses may reduce the capacity to receive emergency admissions.

Duty team

As a consequence of reduced junior doctors' hours without increased numbers, the stage has been reached where the number of patients that has to be looked after by the duty team may be so large that the quality of care may be reduced. Is it reasonable to expect the highest quality of care from a duty team consisting of perhaps three doctors, junior, middle and senior grade, who may be responsible for as many as 150 ill patients? There is a need to examine the number of patients who can be cared for optimally by one small team. I have worked in an 800-bed hospital in Africa as one of only two doctors on duty at night: one for the medical wards, who also did the cross-matching of blood, whilst the other looked after the casualty department and the X-rays. That is a fire-brigade type of service, but we are heading in the same direction in the UK.

Admissions policy

Given that the service for acute G(I)M is demand-led, attempts have been made to control the inflow by restricting the capacity of any particular hospital to absorb acute medical patients. I shall quote the experiences of my own hospital, Newcastle General Hospital, which is a DGH and teaching hospital serving the west end of Newcastle, a fairly socially deprived area.[1] The buildings are largely 19th century, based on the old workhouse (a name still applied affectionately by those working within it, and derogatorily by those working in newer hospitals elsewhere in the city). The lack of a roof over the patients' heads as they move from one part of the site to another belies the good reputation which the hospital has of caring for its patients.

The hospital used to have a tradition of which it was proud, which may be encapsulated in the expression 'we never closed'. This policy, which was operative until the mid-1980s, was that any patient requiring admission would be found a bed somewhere in the hospital until not a single empty bed was left. In practice, this meant that patients in the convalescent stage would move from ward to ward to vacate more appropriate beds on the acute receiving wards. This resulted in legitimate complaints when relatives could not find their loved ones on the ward where they had been yesterday and feared they might have gone 'upstairs', before finding they had been moved down the corridor or into another block. More seriously, such a policy impinged gravely on the work of other departments, particularly the surgical departments whose operating lists were cancelled, and whose waiting lists grew longer because the beds were occupied by acutely ill medical rather than surgical patients.

The disruption this caused resulted in a change of philosophy, whereby it was determined that boarding patients out of their appropriate medical ward should be reduced to a minimum. This could be achieved only by deflecting GP referrals to another hospital, provided that the other hospital had the capacity to absorb medical patients. This still left the duty medical officers with the problem of how to absorb the patients who presented to the A&E department. Such patients have to be admitted whenever necessary, and the practice was to board them into whichever ward had sufficient nurses to care for them until another, more appropriate, bed became available in the next day or two.

Interestingly, it was subsequently shown that this policy considerably improved the quality of care and reduced the duration of admissions, resulting in a higher turnover of patients in the 12 months following the procedure than had previously been the case. There was less interference with other departments in the hospital, and patients received better attention because the medical teams were not running all over the hospital trying to find them.

Effects of reduction in bed capacity

A subsequent reduction in the medical bed capacity by approximately 25% to save money due to a reduction in Newcastle's capitation income has had further consequences, some of which could be predicted. The demand for the service from local practitioners and the accident service did not diminish in the 12-month period following the reduction in bed capacity compared with the 12 previous months. The pressure to admit and to discharge patients resulted in a reduced length of stay, which now averages about six days on the medical wards, ranging from one day to more than a month. This should not be considered in isolation from the turnover interval which has been reduced from a few hours to minutes in some cases, a process known as 'hot-bedding'.

The duration of stay is of course related to the age, medical con-

dition and social circumstances of the patients. The hospital oper-
ates a combined acute medicine/geriatric service, whereby patients
of any age are admitted to the acute medical wards and to such
beds as are available on the geriatric wards. It is of interest to note
that the median age of the medical (that is, non-geriatric) patients
is about 65, which means that half the patients admitted are over
this age, and the median age in the geriatric wards is about 80.
Social support (or rather the lack of it) often determines how long
the patient will actually stay in the ward. An improved rehabilitation
service could result in shorter stays on the acute wards.

Whilst the quantity of activities per bed has increased, it is more
questionable whether the quality of the services has been maintained. There have been increased complaints from patients, who
are usually moved at least once, if not twice, during any admission
from the acute ward to another ward when a bed is not initially
available on the base ward of the admitting team.

There have also been increased complaints from GPs who cannot get their patients admitted. This concern is shared by the hospital medical staff, particularly when they are unable to accept
their own patients back again. It is not in the best interests of
patients to be sent to another hospital rather than the one where
they are already known, and which may well have discharged them
only the previous week.

The staff feel continuously under pressure. Running any system
to its maximum capacity does not make for optimal performance.
There is not enough flexibility to cope with the variations in
demand for medical beds, and boarding patients into inappropriate departments results.

Cost constraints

Furthermore, because the activities have been increased, the costs
have also increased. No further funding is forthcoming, although
the 3% margin over the block contract has been exceeded. The
hospital is thus predicted to overspend for the financial year. If
additional funding cannot be provided, and if business principles
are to be applied, the purchasing authority should limit the number of patients with access to the service. Once referrals have been
made, however, there is a responsibility ethically and medicolegally
to provide care, backed up by facilities which conform to an
acceptable standard. The use of suboptimal clinical protocols is
clearly indefensible. The options are rather stark: if the cost cannot be met, should more medical beds be closed and fewer nurses

employed? At the same time, how can boarding into other specialties' beds be prevented? Should the hospital close to all medical
emergencies when the budget is spent?

General effects of reduced bed capacity in the NHS

The example given above might be thought of as special pleading for
a particular situation in one hospital, but this experience is not
unique. Petty and Gumpel compared the acute medical admission
patterns in similar periods over three consecutive years, between the
first and second of which a sudden reduction in acute bed numbers
took place, at Northwick Park Hospital.[2] The results showed that the
hospital was closed to admissions from GPs on three out of 25 days in
the first year, but on 20 out of 31 days by the third year. Not surpris-
ingly, the number of patients referred by the GPs fell from 56% to
44%, but the number of self-referred patients admitted via the A&E
department rose from 27% to 39%. Furthermore, an increasing proportion of the patients admitted were elderly, representing 25% of
admissions in 1986, but 44% in 1988. The increasing age of the population and the needs of the elderly for the acute medical services
are placing increased demand on a service with a reduced capacity.

The Tomlinson Report

The recent Tomlinson Report on the hospital scene in London
expressed the efficiency of bed usage in terms of the number of
beds used per 1,000 episodes of acute care.[3] An average of 20
beds/1,000 episodes for all hospital activities is deemed to be relatively inefficient, and a target of 10 beds/1,000 acute episodes is
thought to be desirable. When these figures are applied to acute
medical wards they are equivalent to an average length of stay
being reduced from approximately one week (one bed for 50
episodes/year) to half a week per patient. It is difficult to see how
this can be achieved for acute general medical patients, given the
wide range of their conditions. Thus, a patient with an uncomplicated heart attack may need only a few days to recover, whereas
someone with a stroke may need more than a month,

Day-case care

Day-case care is equivalent to an efficiency rating of approximately
three beds/1,000 episodes (one bed/330 episodes) if one patient
episode occurs per bed every day of the year except Sundays and

Bank Holidays. This is a useful figure, based on models of surgical care or day-case investigations, but it is not applicable to emergency medical admissions. There is a danger that in the laudable drive for efficiency, a lack of understanding of the different nature of medical and surgical models of care will result in resources being squeezed to a level below that required to meet the legitimate needs of the acutely ill population.

Optimum conditions for an acute medical service

The question which has to be addressed is: What are the optimum conditions required to maintain an acute medical service? The need for the acute services is not always being met, and the capacity to respond to it should not be reduced to such a level whereby it is commonplace to send a patient to another city 10 or 20 miles away. The quality of care for those who are admitted must not fall below acceptable standards.

Coping with the acute demands on the service is one of the most stressful experiences any hospital doctor can undergo in his/her training. A great deal of the stress is caused not by the complexity of the patient's problems but by trying to find a bed in an appropriate place where the patient can be properly nursed and cared for. Long hours are not the only factor contributing to loss of morale amongst junior doctors.

Solutions can be found if plans are based on optimal rather than maximum bed usage. Bed usage should be geared to leave a margin of capacity to cope with the day-to-day fluctuations in demand. This capacity should be planned to let the hospital absorb, say, up to 95% of the day-to-day variation in acute admissions. There will inevitably be occasions when the number of admissions required still exceeds one hospital's bed capacity. Major epidemics or wars do not pose problems because the hospital can close down elective work to cope with the resulting huge surge in demand. Witness the preparations made in anticipation of the return of large numbers of casualties from the Gulf War, which fortunately were not required.

Such solutions are of course drastic; they markedly impinge on other proper hospital activities and add to waiting lists. Some reserve capacity is however needed to cope with the less drastic but predictable surges in demand for the service, particularly in the winter months.

Here it may be worth drawing an analogy with the planning that occurs in the power industry. Most coal-fired power stations work most efficiently at a steady production rate, which can provide 90%

of the power requirements of the population for most of the time. These power stations cannot, however, cope with the sudden surge in demand when everybody puts on their electric kettle at half-time during the World Cup or similar events. This sudden demand for power is met by releasing reserves of energy stored within the mountains of Wales or Scotland in the form of high reservoirs. The water is pumped up at night from low reservoirs at relatively cheap times, and released to drive turbines which can cope with the demand at peak times. Similar foresight in planning is needed in the health service to provide the reserves to cope with the needs. The acute service in many hospitals is now overstretched and fails at times of stress.

Conclusions

In summary, the services for acute G(I)M are demand-led. There are no waiting lists and negligible elective work. Referrals to hospitals are seldom inappropriate and hospitals should not turn away needy, ill people who arrive on their doorstep. Deflection of GP referrals elsewhere is increasing, which is unsatisfactory for all concerned and also leads to increased unreferred admissions via the A&E department.

Reduction of lengths of stay with improved social support in the community may improve the efficiency of bed usage, but older patients take longer to heal. Reduction of bed capacity ahead of any reduction in demand leads to increased boarding out of patients on inappropriate wards, knock-on effects on other departments, and interference with their elective work, which adds to waiting lists.

Whilst there has to be a ceiling on the level of service that can be provided, it should be high enough to cope with at least 95% of the variation in daily demand. Plans to bring reserve facilities into use to cope with predictable extra demand, such as occurs in winter, should be ready to be put into operation at short notice.

If the provider units (the hospitals) fail to fulfil their contractual obligations, they need to say why they failed, and the purchaser (still the health authority for most acute medical services) has the right to place a contract elsewhere. Where the provider unit fulfils its contract but the needs of the population for the acute services are still not being met, the purchasers have the responsibility to explain and to rectify any shortfall. If the required level of service cannot be met, the reasons should be made explicit. The term 'rationing' acknowledges that there are limitations, but also implies that a reasonable approach has been made to ensure adequate provision for the acutely ill and their needs.

References

1.   Townsend P, Davidson N, eds. *Inequalities in health: the Black Report.* London: Penguin Books, 1982.
2.   Petty R, Gumpel M. Acute medical admissions: changes following a sudden reduction in bed numbers at Northwick Park Hospital. *Journal of the Royal College of Physicians* 1990; **24:** 32–5.
3.   *Inquiry into London's health service, medical education and research: the Tomlinson Report.* London: HMSO, 1992.

5 | Health care rationing and elderly people

John Grimley Evans
Professor of Geriatric Medicine, Department of Clinical Geratology, Radcliffe Infirmary, Oxford

Health care resources are limited. This undeniable fact is sometimes presented as if it were a great given of the universe before which politicians and administrators are of necessity powerless and prostrate. This is to overstate the case. As a nation, we are probably rich enough to provide a health service that could meet all reasonable demands. The bottomless bucket of health demands is a convenient myth for those who have never seriously tried to fill the bucket.

In the field of geriatric medicine, there was much concern in the 1970s about the general inadequacy of geriatric services. It was apparent, however, that services regarded by professionals and public alike as entirely sufficient were being provided in a small number of districts in England. Study showed that this was being achieved at levels of resource that were undoubtedly above the national average but not inaccessibly above.[1]

The limits on health care that determine the degree of necessary rationing are imposed by, and are the responsibility of, government. Quite properly, government has to decide how little is to be made available for public spending from taxation, and how much it will allocate to the health care of the population, compared with what is to be spent in other areas such as defence or social security payments for the unemployed. While it is our duty as citizens and professionals to take part in implementing systems of rationing made necessary by government policies, these activities should not be allowed to distract us or the public we serve from remembering that one way of reducing the impact of rationing would be for a government to increase the health budget. The rationing of health care is contingent on a higher level of rationing decisions between different national priorities, and this fact should be retained in the debate.

Rationing and equity

The concept of rationing has a number of aspects. When discussed in the context of health care, the main preoccupation seems often to be rationing in the sense of restriction. During the Second World War rationing in Britain acquired the additional and beneficent implication of equitable distribution. Most of us will be committed to the view that the issue of equity must remain central and explicit in the application of rationing to the publicly funded health and social services in Britain. The ability of the rich to buy for themselves things which are to be denied to the poor is a matter that needs to be held in mind, but we should not fall into the trap of assuming that the rich are always wise in their purchasing, or necessarily benefit from it. Many geriatricians have derived comfort over the years from a comparison of National Health Service (NHS) and the independent sector of health care which has demonstrated that important aspects of care for older people in the NHS are better than those purchasable in the private market. Even among those professionally committed exclusively to the public sector few would wish to see a state monopoly of the health care market.

If equity is to be maintained, it will need to be visible, which implies that the basis of rationing should be made public and explicit. Doctors should not arrogate to themselves the task of rationing, which should remain and be clearly seen to be the responsibility of the public's elected representatives. Rationing should not be allowed to take place by cutting quality or fudging eligibility criteria. If the government and its servants in the purchasing authorities consider that they are able only to buy x operations when $x + n$ people need them, the value of n must be a matter of public knowledge and comment. No democratically mandated government could wish otherwise.

Rationing and the ageing population

Issues of health care rationing have an especial impact on elderly people. One reason is the ageing of the population, and the particular increase in the numbers and proportions of the very old. Health and social care expenditures show a U-shaped relationship with age: among the most expensive things an individual can do is to be born and to be a child, but average expenditures fall thereafter to rise again over the years past middle age.[2] The ageing of the British population is already well advanced compared with some other nations such as the USA and Canada. Although it will continue into the next century, the implications for costs over that period are not as great as is often assumed. Recent estimates, for example, suggest that if provision remains at present levels health service costs attributable to population ageing will only be of the order of 5% in hospital and community sector costs, and 3% in general practitioner (GP) and prescription costs over the present decade. The growth in institutional care costs will be much greater at around 17%.[2] For various reasons, it is to be hoped that the age pattern of provision should not remain as at present, in particular with rather more spent on health interventions in old age and rather less on institutional care. Present levels of provision may be excessive due to distortion by the recent uncontrolled expansion of the private nursing home industry. The overall effect of such desirable care changes on costs is uncertain but not necessarily great.

Ageism in medicine

A further reason why rationing is a salient issue in considering health care for older people is that they are already the victims of restrictions on care that are not applied to other age groups. In the USA, there is evidence that the contact between older people and their doctors is less than proportional to the prevalence of disorders meriting consultation and to their additional history and sometimes slower communication.[3] Ageism has been abundantly documented in the USA in the field of cancer, for which older people are less likely to be offered potentially curative care.[4,5]

In Britain, ageist discrimination has been documented in the management of renal failure. Wing pointed out that only 8% of patients offered renal dialysis were over 65, compared with around 25% in Germany, France and Italy.[6] This cannot be justified in terms of response to the treatment. Taube *et al.* have shown a 62% five-year survival in people aged 65 and over, compared with 44% in patients aged 55–64 in pooled European data.[7] Data from Oxford have suggested that the quality of life enjoyed by older patients on peritoneal dialysis is no less than that of younger patients.[8] The problem, as Taube and colleagues pointed out, may be partly that the doctors considering referral of elderly patients, notably GPs, do not know enough about modern nephrology.[7] Fund-holding GPs of the future may have other reasons for not referring patients for nephrological care.

Ageist bias has also emerged in studies of cardiological interventions. Elder *et al.* showed that older patients coming to coronary angiography were iller than young people, and more often had to undergo emergency rather than elective surgery.[9] Despite this, results of interventions were good, with only a 5% difference in survival rates between young and old patients. The implication seemed to be that older patients were not being referred as readily as the young.

Recent data from the UK on the availability of good quality acute care for myocardial infarction present an even more worrying picture. Despite the pronouncement by a working party of the Royal College of Physicians that there are no clinical grounds for restricting cardiological interventions on the grounds of age alone,[10] Dudley and Burns found that 19% of coronary care units have an upper age limit for admission and 40% have an upper limit for thrombolytic therapy.[11] There is at present no scientific evidence to support these policies.

It seems clear that older people are at risk of being offered inadequate or second-rate treatment simply because they are old. This is the classical condition of 'aggravated ageing'.[12] Old people are expected to do badly, so it is not noticed that they are doing worse than they need because of the poor quality care they are offered.

Science and ageism

Insofar as there could be a clinical rationale for age discrimination, it is that older people are less likely to benefit than younger people. There is widespread misunderstanding of the relationship between age and outcome from health interventions. There is no way in which age, which is no more than a set of numbers on a birth certificate, could directly affect outcomes but it is a common 'category error' for people to speak, write and, alas, even think as if it could. It is the physiological impairments that increase in prevalence with age that produce the average decline in quality of outcome from medical interventions. However, individuals vary greatly in the rate at which their physiology changes with age and, to be scientific, we should be concerned with the physiology of patients not their age. Indeed, if age remains in a predictive equation after feeding in all the available data specifying an individual's physiological status and reserve, we have either failed to measure all the relevant variables or measured them inaccurately. Moreover, as Manolio and Furberg point out, if age does remain in the predictive equation, it would be logical for this to be regarded as an indicator of a need for extra care and surveillance, not as an excuse for withholding care.[13]

Not enough systematic clinical and physiological research has been done to provide the basis for individualised risk/benefit predictions for even the commonest interventions. It is rather disgraceful that this work has not been done, but the new arrangements for research and development instituted by the Department of Health offer an unprecedented opportunity for the systematic data collection that could start to provide the desired answers. If individualised risk/benefit predictions could be made, we may suspect that more old people in Britain than at present would undergo beneficial interventions. The costs would be balanced to some extent by some younger people being spared predictably futile interventions to which they are unthinkingly subjected simply because they are young.

There is a further area of care for elderly people where rationing needs a more scientific rationale. One of the first established principles of good geriatric medicine was that no one should be consigned to the status of high dependency or placed in an institution until a trial of rehabilitation by an appropriately skilled team had been undertaken. This may no longer be a feasible policy given its costs and manpower implications. Some kind of rational triage system is needed to save patients both from unnecessary institutionalisation and from unproductive attempts at rehabilitation. This would release staff and other resources to provide more intensive, and therefore more rapidly effective, therapy to those who will benefit.

Again, the problem is that there are not the systematic data to provide a rational basis for such triage, and again we would like to see the new information structures in the NHS used to answer such questions.

The ethics of ageism

The ethical issues of ageism are less easily dealt with. In the USA, the effectiveness of older people in using their voting power to obtain more health and social resources has alarmed advocates for other social groups who feel disadvantaged by the transfer of resources to the old. No transfer of comparable size has occurred in Britain. The USA problem may be redefinable: it may not be that the old have been given too much, but that the *total* amount to give is too low owing to government restrictions on public spending.

Be that as it may, there is now a brisk business in the development and marketing of reasons for restricting the access of the old and poor to health care. Daniel Callahan is particularly prominent among the ethicists engaged in this debate. He has taken up a concept of natural lifespan as:

> the achievement of a life long enough to accomplish for the most part those opportunities that life typically affords people and which we ordinarily take to be the prime benefits of life . . .[14]

As clinicians, we would not quarrel with the existential concept of natural lifespan that this definition seems to imply. We all see patients who have reached the end both of their body's capacity and their mind's appetite for survival, who have achieved all that has for them been possible, for whom desire is suspended and hope extinguished, and all without regret. This is a state we recognise and honour, and to which in due course we must ourselves submit. However, a few lines on, Callahan's experiential concept of natural lifespan has slid into something which has the same name but is fundamentally different, a lifespan defined by age:

> My own view is that it can now be achieved by the late 70s or early 80s.[14]

From this, Callahan goes on to say that under 'public entitlement programs' beyond the natural lifespan

> government should provide only the means necessary for the relief of suffering not life-extending technology.

I cannot identify the ideological basis for this ethical stance with what I have long assumed to be that of British and American society.[15]

Quality of life

In this country, discrimination against the old is rationalised not by ethicists but by economists who are being increasingly called upon to justify patterns of priorities within the health services. The institutionalisation of ageism in the British health system could be consolidated by the use of indices correlated with duration of survival, such as quality-adjusted life years (QALYs) to determine resource allocation.

The ethical basis of the QALY as a means of allocating resources between different people (as distinct from helping an individual to choose between different treatments for his or her disease) has been generally criticised by several authors.[16] There are some specific and unsolved technical problems with the QALY that could increase its discriminatory effect against older people, and different ways of measuring quality of life that are not necessarily equivalent. The psychometric approach is to ask individuals to give an overall impression of their quality of life or how they would value a state of existence presented to them in descriptive form. In the functional approach, the activities of which an individual is capable might be counted, with the assumption that quality of life deteriorates progressively with increasing numbers of disabilities.

These two approaches, although both loosely called quality of life, are clearly different and there is evidence to suggest that confusion between the two can foster ageist discrimination against older people. For example, there is an interesting literature relating to old people's wishes about cardiopulmonary resuscitation when they are admitted to hospitals or nursing homes. The data show that, in general, more old people wish for invasive care of various types, including cardiopulmonary resuscitation, than is assumed not only by the doctors and nurses looking after them but also by the old people's relatives.[17]

These findings are worrying, because explicit or implicit proxy decisions are commonly made on behalf of older people. One likely reason why relatives and medical health attendants underestimate old people's desire for life prolongation is a confusion between the two types of assessment of quality of life. An outside observer is likely to weight patients' quality of life by their perceived functional status. Old people themselves, however, will judge their quality of life by their general sense of enjoyment, and they can psychologically adjust even to quite severe physical disabilities.

One approach to the uncertainty about who should decide on the weighting factors for QALYs has been the suggestion that, since the general public pays for the NHS, it would be appropriate to solicit their views about the weighting factors to be used. This is of course the basis of the Oregon experiment.[18] In an experiment in Cardiff, a sample of the public were asked to state which of two patients they would wish to be treated if there were treatment available only for one.[19,20] The findings of the study showed that, in general, the public placed highest value upon lives of older children versus younger children and on younger adults versus older adults. The authors of the report point out that this reflects ageist prejudices, but suggest that because it expresses the views of the public it may be appropriate for ageist prejudices to be built into the system.

There were two things wrong with this experiment: first, that it did not offer the respondents the choice of tossing a coin to decide which of two people had the treatment. Professor John Harris and others have pointed out that random allocation is the most equitable way of distributing limited resources, but the average man in the Cardiff street will be unlikely to think of this for himself.

Secondly, in order to work out the full implications of what they were about, the investigators should have made the questionnaire confidential and offered a control choice between a black patient and a white patient, or even a Welshman and an Englishman. If that had revealed (as would not have been surprising) a degree of racism in the general public of Cardiff, would the authors then have suggested that it would be reasonable to build racism into the system of provision of health care in this country? I suspect not—and a plea that the difference is that racism is illegal but ageism is not could surely only be urged by the morally destitute.

The fallacy underlying this approach is that the rights of individual citizens should be put into the hands of other citizens. The rights of an individual should be embodied in the constitution of the state, whether that constitution is written or implicit. One of the principles of the British state is that all citizens are equal in having equal status before the law and equal basic access to the means of life, education and health. People are not made less equal because of their skin colour or their sex, and it is not appropriate to make them less equal because of height, eye colour, age or any other biological variable over which the individual can have no control. Such rights should not be withdrawn from the citizens of this country by any means other than formal Act of Parliament.

The customers and the shopkeepers

An argument can also be made against QALYs as being a purveyor's rather than a customer's measure of outcome. Some people might be prepared to argue that because a person of 80 has a lower life expectancy than someone of 50, the state somehow gets less for its money from treating an older person than from treating a younger one. There are several things wrong with this argument. First, in the individual case it may not be true. If surgery makes the difference between the old person returning to live independently in his or her own home rather than surviving for many years disabled in a nursing home (a possible outcome from withholding heart surgery for angina, for example), it is economically a good investment. Furthermore, a person aged 50 needing heart surgery is unlikely to be physiologically a good specimen, and his chances may not be good of living out the average lifespan for a 50-year-old. In any case, is it appropriate to let what the state as purveyor gets from the health services determine what the patient as customer is offered? Does the taxpayer see himself as a shareholder in a chain of health shops or as a customer of a health service? We have perhaps allowed ourselves to slip too easily into the fast talk of the market-place without stopping to think whether we wish to be the buyers or the sellers.

The market provides a realistic model for health care only if it can be forged into a theoretically perfect market. There are at least two features of the perfect market that are not yet in place: first, there must be genuine choice, which there is not, and second, the customers should be sophisticated customers, or 'good consumers'.[21] They must know what could be available, and be able and prepared to demand the best. If there is no genuine choice and customers do not know what to demand, the market functions merely as a device for exploiting the customer. Even in the USA, where the gods of the market-place have long been worshipped, the particular vulnerability of the older health service customer is recognised.[3]

The differing objectives of the customers and of the purveyors of health services need to be kept constantly in mind as we join in the development of the new NHS. Despite its obvious virtues, there is a provocative paradox in the purchaser/provider split of the new NHS. The paradox is that the traditional advocates for the unsophisticated customer, the doctors, nurses and other caring professionals who encounter on a daily basis the needs of the suffering, and on whom such suffering places a direct moral and palpable responsibility, will be classified with the providers, while the official purchasers, those who will be presented as serving the interests of the customer, will be the servants and placemen of the purveyors in central government. Perhaps what has been called the 'glorious ungovernability of the English' will defend us from the hazards of this alarming example of Orwellian Newspeak. Even more Orwellian is the idea that citizens' access to specialist health care should be through fund-holding GPs whose profits will be the greater the more they manage to prevent such access.

An opportunity from scarcity

Many treatments now offered have never been properly evaluated, but because they are in general use it is considered unethical to subject them to randomised controlled trials. If rationing is made sufficiently explicit, it offers an opportunity to carry out randomised controlled trials of withholding treatment since, as has already been noted, the most equitable way of distributing limited resources is by random allocation. This opportunity of scarcity was exploited to carry out a successful randomised controlled trial of rehousing as a means of improving mental health.[22] If this example were followed systematically, the cloud of rationing might be found to have a silver lining in the scope for redeployment of currently wasted resources.

Envoi

Before we start rationing we must start being rational, and there are scientific and ethical issues to be settled. Older people are citizens, and should be treated as such in whatever system of rationing is eventually decided upon. With regard to that, I suspect (to steal from T. S. Eliot) that the end of all our exploring will be to arrive where we started—in an orderly old-fashioned British queue.

References

1. Grimley Evans J. Hospital care for the elderly. In: Shegog REA, ed. *The impending crisis of old age.* Oxford: Nuffield Provincial Hospitals Trust, 1981: 133–46.
2. The Association of the British Pharmaceutical Industry. *Agenda for health 1991. The challenges of ageing.* London: ABPI, 1991.
3. Kane RA, Kane RL. Self-care and health care: inseparable but equal for the wellbeing of the old. In: Dean K, Hickey T, Holstein BE, eds. *Self-care and health in old age.* London: Croom Helm, 1986: 251–83.
4. Samet J, Hunt WC, Key C, Humble CG, Goodwin JS. Choice of cancer therapy varies with age of patient. *Journal of the American Medical Association* 1986; **255**: 3385–90.
5. Greenfield S, Blanco DM, Elashoff RM, Ganz PA. Patterns of care related to age of breast cancer patients. *Journal of the American Medical Association* 1987; **257**: 2766–70.
6. Wing AJ. Why don't the British treat more patients with kidney failure? *British Medical Journal* 1984; **287**: 1157–8.
7. Taube DH, Winder EA, Ogg CS, Bewick M, Cameron JS, Rudge CJ, Williams DG. Successful treatment of middle-aged and elderly patients with end-stage renal disease. *British Medical Journal* 1983; **286**: 2018–20.
8. Winearls CG, Oliver DO, Auer J. Age and dialysis. *Lancet* 1992; **339**: 432.
9. Elder AT, Shaw TRD, Turnbull CM, Starkey IR. Elderly and younger patients selected to undergo coronary angiography. *British Medical Journal* 1991; **303**: 950–3.
10. A report of a working group of the Royal College of Physicians. Cardiological interventions in elderly patients. *Journal of the Royal College of Physicians* 1991; **25**: 197–205.

11. Dudley NJ, Burns E. The influence of age on policies for admission and thrombolysis in coronary care units in the United Kingdom. *Age and Ageing* 1992; **21**: 95–8.
12. Grimley Evans J. The biology of human ageing. In: Dawson AM, Compston N, Besser GM, eds. *Recent advances in medicine, No. 18*. London: Churchill Livingstone, 1981: 17–37.
13. Manolio TA, Furberg CD. Age as a predictor of outcome: what role does it play? *American Journal of Medicine* 1992; **92**: 1–6.
14. Callahan D. Aging and the ends of medicine. *Annals of the New York Academy of Sciences* 1988; **530**: 125–32.
15. Grimley Evans J. Age and equality. *Annals of the New York Academy of Sciences* 1988; **530**: 118–24.
16. Harris J. QALYfying the value of life. *Journal of Medical Ethics* 1987; **13**: 117–23.
17. Seckler AB, Meier DE, Mulvihill M, Cammer Paris BE. Substituted judgement: how accurate are proxy predictions? *Annals of Internal Medicine* 1991; **115**: 92–8.
18. Chapter 2, this volume.
19. Lewis PA, Charny M. Which of two individuals do you treat when only their ages are different and you cannot treat both? *Journal of Medical Ethics* 1989; **15**: 28–32.
20. Charny M, Lewis PA. Choosing who shall be treated in the NHS. *Social Science and Medicine* 1989; **28**: 1331–8.
21. Donaldson C, Lloyd P, Lupton D. Primary health care consumerism amongst elderly Australians. *Age and Ageing* 1991; **20**: 280–6.
22. Elton PJ, Packer JM. A prospective randomised trial of the value of rehousing on the grounds of mental ill-health. *Journal of Chronic Diseases* 1986; **39**: 221–8.

6 | End-stage renal failure

Netar P Mallick

Professor of Renal Medicine, University of Manchester

In the continuing debate on the delivery of health care in Britain other people have been more vocal than the medical profession. Such reticence might indicate an unwillingness to enter into the discussion on an extremely complicated topic. Doctors should welcome the wide interest taken in their work because they are totally dependent on the community they serve. If what doctors can provide is not needed, it need not be provided. On the other hand, doctors are always uniquely placed to assess what is needed through their close involvement with the community they serve. It is questionable whether the medical profession has done enough to define the needs it perceives and to suggest ways in which these can be met. It may be that a hiatus has been left into which others have entered vigorously.

It is not sufficient for the profession to assert that benefit will accrue. The community does not afford such wide delegation of its resources to doctors—rather, their duty is to *demonstrate* the benefit. Even if an individual benefits from an intervention, the consequence of providing *that* intervention for *that* individual patient does not address the total commitment of the community. In equity, each such individual patient should receive the same beneficial intervention, so doctors need to spell out this total commitment in terms of resources needed and benefit gained. A realistic plan for provision could be established only if the sum of all such commitments is available. It need hardly be said that we are far from such a position, yet such data are needed year-on-year to ensure that appropriate resources are made available.

The response of health economists and others has been to seek tools which will require clinicians so to order their approach as to make apparently rational decisions possible about which interventions and in what volume a service should provide. An extension of this approach has been to develop methods which, it is claimed, make it possible for purchasers to assess the relative benefits of disparate interventions and so to choose which (and which not) to provide.

Definition of health and sickness

Central to this approach is the assertion that there is a limit to the resources available for the health service, but no limit to the resources that health care might demand, so that choice is inevitable. I suggest that this is an untested (if widely held) assertion. It is more realistic to address a different question: Can the nation afford to treat the sick? This question both sharpens and clarifies the debate. It concentrates on what really disturbs and frightens people—sickness. 'Sickness' requires definition.

Health and sickness are not two ends of a continuous spectrum. The concept of 'health' is neither fixed nor simple. It subsumes physical, mental and social well-being to a level that might be considered as the acceptable minimum in that society—the health equivalent of a 'minimum wage'—but, however conceived, it is a moving target as aspirations increase in increasingly educated and affluent communities. The perception of what constitutes well-being (health) will always outstrip the resources of any community to provide for every citizen throughout life.

'Illness' may be considered not as a negative state, as the lack of perceived health, but rather as a result of positive events or factors which so distort physical, mental and social well-being as to remove the individual from the rest of the population. This is as valid for minor temporary illness such as a respiratory tract infection as for a serious and permanent one. Serious illness, especially if it is long-lasting, dominates life for the individual and the family, and even minor illness distorts that life temporarily. It is part of the everyday working knowledge of the clinician that this is so, but few others in the community appreciate the dislocating effects of illness unless it strikes them directly.

As in other developed countries, the expansion of demand for the treatment of illness in Britain has been mainly in relation to the ageing population, while the prevention of premature death has focused on the current scourges of cardiovascular, respiratory and neoplastic disease. Only a few other conditions, one of which is renal failure, have become treatable because of technical advances.

If the National Health Service (NHS) is to take seriously its intention to provide, free of charge at the point of delivery, the care needed to prevent premature death for each of its citizens—and, despite cynical views expressed, I believe this is the intention—precise evidence is needed as to what should be provided.

Renal failure as a paradigm for health care

Renal failure is a paradigm of such an approach. The condition is clear-cut: kidneys fail and death ensues. If renal replacement therapy (RRT) is provided, kidney function is substituted sufficiently for premature death to be prevented. Median survival is greater than ten years in patients up to 60 years old at the start of treatment, and remains at over five years for many patients in their 70s. The quality of life has been documented, and the individual is restored to the approximate level of activity formerly enjoyed. Interestingly, the quality of life improves with time as adjustments to the demands of regular treatment are effected.

The number of cases for which the service might need to be provided has been quantified prospectively in the UK. It appears to be stable at 75–80 new patients per million population (pmp) up to age 70, for whom such treatment will both prevent premature death and restore active life, and in whom intercurrent incapacity from other causes will not dominate the outcome. Intercurrent illness influences outcome, as do the pressures on the family of such regular treatment. These influences add quantifiable demands to the services required to treat patients in renal failure. The cost of treatment is well rehearsed. Unit costs for dialysis have fallen dramatically over the past two decades, although advances continually develop.

Thus, the profession has provided all the elements required for the community to assess its responsibilities for the treatment of end-stage renal failure (ESRF). The evidence provided is instructive.

Renal replacement therapy in the UK

Prospective studies were conducted in Scotland, North-West and South-West England, and Northern Ireland (Table 1). These confirmed that overall approximately 80 patients pmp would benefit from RRT. Patients were excluded in whom the complexity of other co-morbid conditions was likely to reduce the value of RRT to that of simply sustaining a hospital-bound or near hospital-bound life until death ensued from another cause. The overall incidence covers wide age-specific differences, both in the rate of incidence and in the cause of the renal failure. The age-specific incidence of ESRF rises sharply in older aged cohorts (Table 2). It

Table 1. Summary of the results of prospective studies on renal replacement therapy in the UK (1982–88).[1]

- 80 patients pmp per year develop end-stage renal failure
- 300 patients pmp will need assessment for renal replacement therapy
  (80 patients needing treatment in that year will come from this cohort)
- an additional 600 patients pmp have established renal impairment, not at end-stage but requiring clinical management and pre-end-stage assessment if optimal results are to be achieved

pmp = per million population

Table 2. Age-related incidence of chronic renal failure in Devon (see reference 1).

Age (years)	% of population	Number at risk	Chronic renal failure	Incidence (pmp/year)
<20	25	111,500	1	9
20–39	26	116,000	14	63
40–49	12	53,500	8	75
50–59	11	49,100	15	158
60–69	12	53,500	22	206
70–79	9	40,100	33	412
80+	5	35,700	36	504

pmp = patients per million population

is clear that the present figures represent a substantial and sustained shortfall in the provision of RRT for new patients in the UK, with a consequent low stock of patients on treatment (Table 3). In other European countries of equivalent size and development, most patients who need RRT receive it.[1] This is not so in the UK.

The balance of RRT in the UK is strongly orientated to transplantation and to continuous ambulatory peritoneal dialysis (CAPD). Both are highly effective treatments, but the latter requires centre haemodialysis back-up for patients with intercurrent illness or in whom the treatment has failed. Centre haemodialysis close to home is also needed for many socially and physically vulnerable patients. The figures show that this is significantly underprovided in the UK. Although the UK service is deficient in its overall provision of RRT, it is efficient in utilising as far as possible the more cost-effective modes of treatment (Table 4).

The few doctors available for this specialty (including accredited senior registrars not yet in consultant post) are no more than 120

Table 3. Renal replacement therapy: new entrants and stock (per million population).

Country	New entrants	Stock
UK	63	370
France	77	417
Germany (W)	94	439*
Italy	85	570

* Data precede the unification of Germany.

Table 4. Treatment modalities (%).

Treatment	UK	France	Germany (W)	Italy
Home haemodialysis	6	6	2	2
Continuous ambulatory peritoneal dialysis	22	6	5	8
Centre haemodialysis	17	60	70	74
Transplantation	55	28	22	18

whole-time equivalent doctors for 58 million people (2 pmp) and, together with the few centres available (less than 2 pmp) act as a rationing mechanism. Staffing recommendations for the UK to support the take-on rate of 70–80 patients pmp are shown in Table 5. By comparison, in Italy and France there are some 20 and 15 doctors pmp, respectively, and approximately eight centres pmp in both countries. These figures suggest a doctor/patient ratio of about 100 per whole-time equivalent in the UK, compared to 28 in Italy and 29 in France. Even allowing for the structural differences in health care provision in different European countries, these figures, taken together, are either an indictment of the British approach to the provision of health care, or require a closely analysed debate about

Table 5. Staffing implications (for further details see Ref. 2).

Consultants	
Recommended level:	330 physicians
Current level:	110 physicians
Junior medical staff	
Nursing staff	
Technical, dietetic and social support	

the philosophy on which that health care provision is determined.

The lack of nephrologists in many parts of the country has a perhaps underappreciated negative effect on the efficiency, quality and cost-effectiveness (inevitably interlinked concepts) with which care is provided. The nature of progressive renal failure, whatever its primary cause, is to be clinically silent in many cases until end-stage is reached. It is increasingly evident that good management in the pre-renal phase has a major impact on the benefit of RRT and minimises both mortality and morbidity once such replacement therapy is established. This applies to the major problems of hypertension and its consequences of cardiovascular disease, of metabolic bone disease, and also to the problems of adjustment by the patient and family to treatment.

Myocardial infarction is increasingly common in the older cohorts of ESRF patients. It is much less common in Italy, for instance, compared with the UK, but in both countries there is a similar increase in age-specific incidence compared to the general population (Fig. 1). Early assessment pre-ESRF enables identification of patients at risk. However, many cases of early renal failure are missed, and fail to reach a nephrologist before end-stage: 30–40% of patients in many British centres are seen at the end-stage when no other management is possible. This can be improved only if there are earlier opportunities for nephrologists

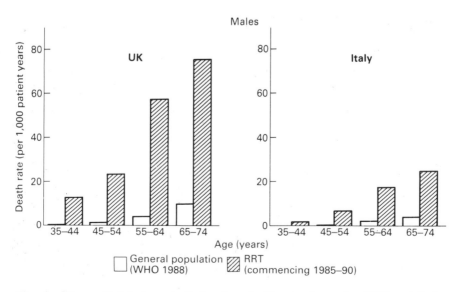

Fig. 1. *Myocardial ischaemia/infarction death rates in males (UK and Italy, 1985–90).*

to assess these patients, but would clearly be cost-effective in terms of timing of transplantation and of any intervention to reduce later morbidity and mortality.

Overall survival is good, so the treatment of a given number of new cases each year necessarily results in an increase in the stock of cases until such time that the death rate from that stock balances the intake rate. This point has not yet been reached in Britain, and is not likely to be achieved for some time.

Quality of life on renal replacement therapy

Quality of life actually improves over the early years. Initially, treatment is a tremendous dislocation of personal and family life with its open-ended commitment both to the discipline of regular, often self-provided treatment, and to restriction on food and fluid intake, hygiene and mobility. Minor disruptions in treatment are common in the early years. Furthermore, it is clear that in these early years pre-existing degenerative illness (especially cardiovascular disease) takes a toll. This is a lesson in itself of the benefits which accrue when patients are seen by a nephrologist early enough in their illness for such problems to be addressed.

Cost profile of renal replacement therapy

The cost profile is instructive. For any new technique there appears to be a biphasic pattern. Initially, the unit costs of treatment are high because technical innovation has high start-up costs, and also because any new intervention is labour-intensive. With time, the cost of each element diminishes, but there is a superimposed volume-associated cost as the potential of the technique is assessed and it is offered to all the patients who might benefit.

RRT is a good example of this cost profile. The cost of disposable equipment needed for a single haemodialysis is currently about £15, whereas it was about £30 15 years ago *without* taking inflation into account. Nursing requirements and nurse/patient ratios have diminished substantially in that time, and the length of each treatment session has been halved. These massive changes in the unit cost of treatment are obscured both by continuing new developments which superimpose their own profile on treatment costs and by the costs incurred in treating patients who, over the years in which they have received RRT, have developed other diseases, or have lost social independence—or who commenced RRT with some of these important, but not disqualifying, disabilities.

Management of end-stage renal failure as a model for other forms of therapy

A highly technical subject such as RRT is a good example of the difficulties that professional and lay people have in understanding together the management of patients with end-stage renal failure. Nephrologists have developed a number of techniques to treat end-stage renal failure. Terms such as haemodialysis, haemodiafiltration, high-flux or biocompatible filters, CAPD are used freely, but they are bewildering to people who are not actually involved. Attempts to reduce so complex a provision into a model applicable to many other forms of treatment of disease are clearly difficult, but health economists have felt the need to attempt this.

The quality-adjusted life year concept

The quality-adjusted life year (QALY) has been used to try to measure the 'value' both of RRT and of its constituent parts. The concept brings together two separate elements in a way which, it is claimed, will make calculable the value of any given treatment with any other treatment, irrespective of its intention and the nature of the disease under consideration: annual financial cost is calculated, an assessment of the quality of life made, and the number of years of likely survival assessed. An adjusting factor is calculated from these three variables for a year of perfect health.

This concept seeks to circumscribe costs, the effective treatment for the individual, and a community-derived value judgement on the worth of the therapy in terms of quality of life it affords to those who receive it. It is not, however, as objective as it appears. Further, it presupposes that the community can decide in each instance, by the use of a few selected and relatively simple parameters, whether a given treatment has 'worth', leaving aside issues particular to the individual. It also assumes that year-on-year the quality of life is static for every patient. This latter assumption is clearly not correct in RRT, in which physical and psychological adjustment in the uncomplicated case makes the treatment over time increasingly smooth for patient and family. Many patients on RRT return to essentially normal working life.

Importantly, RRT fills a nearly unique role in modern medicine. When it is used, life is prolonged; without it, death occurs promptly. In RRT the primary gain for the patient, the family and the community is that the patient lives and can return to his or her normal activity. For most procedures undertaken in the NHS, the gain is not of life itself but rather, for example, improvement of sight in cataract surgery, pain-free mobility in hip replacement, or the relief of severe angina by successful coronary artery reconstruction or dilatation.

Is the quality of life offered by these disparate procedures for disparate illness directly comparable in an objective way? There are wide individual differences which confound an easy assessment of the benefit that each can offer. At the extreme, the benefit of cataract surgery is greater for the healthy alert individual than for one with advanced dementia, and an effective hip replacement will offer greater quality of life to an otherwise fit person than to one with an incapacitating emphysema.

A claim by doctors that treatment is essential to sustain life is compelling, but not sufficient without explanation as to *what* life is sustained. Maintaining life in a highly supportive hospital environment is of limited value if the individual has no prospects of a return to independent activity or cannot utilise the limited potential of a bedridden life. The aim of RRT is to restore sufficient independence for that individual to return to his or her previous life-style with as little intervention as possible. This aim is usually achieved, as has been demonstrated recently by the combined study of the Renal Association and the York Institute of Health Economics.[3]

Cost considerations of the treatment of end-stage renal failure

Cost is an essential—indeed integral—consideration. The costs of RRT are themselves complex. Technical measures, the staff required and the drugs needed must all be considered, as must the cost of supportive surgery which may be required. There is a regular requirement for dietitians, social workers and often psychologists or psychiatrists too. The needs of the family have to be considered constantly, and patients on independent dialysis in the home need regular monitoring by home visiting nurses.

Conclusions

All these points have been well rehearsed. Nevertheless, it has clearly been demonstrated that RRT is effective, that patients may return to their independent lives with a quality equivalent to that of the general population, and that across the lifespan, including the elderly, adjustment to treatment can be extremely good. Natural lifespan is not extended, however, and in the elderly survival reflects the *other* disabilities of the aged.

The social deprivation that ESRF produces in those without a supportive family is not addressed sufficiently. Structured social support would add to the quality which can be provided by the treatment.

The British form of health care to which the community is so committed is quite different from an insurance-based system in which the individual is required to make a judgement as to what health care is to be provided.

The QALY concept may have a role in assessing the relative benefit of treatment for comparable diseases where the aim is to improve well-being, but otherwise it introduces an approach of 'central decision making by non-clinical parameters, diminishing rather than enhancing both the right to, and the choice of, treatment for individuals. A much better approach for the NHS would be to establish a true hierarchy of treatment provision, in which those treatments which aim both to sustain life and to maintain for the individual his or her otherwise existing quality of life must rank at the top. Those treatments which reverse illness or remove disability rank higher than those which simply restore well-being. Such an easily understood and, I suspect, readily acceptable hierarchy would leave the QALY concept with a role *within* these agreed groups rather than *across* them.

A scale of disability and the cost of treatment are essential parts of the evaluation of medical management but overzealously to link them is to introduce a novel, even mischievous, framework for the treatment of illness.

References

1. Feest TG, Mistry CD, Grimes DS, Mallick NP. Incidence of advanced chronic renal failure and the need for end-stage renal replacement treatment. *British Medical Journal* 1990; **301:** 897–900.
2. Renal Association. *Provision of services for adult patients with renal disease in the UK.* Working group report. London: Renal Association and Royal College of Physicians, 1991.
3. de Charro FTh, Feest TG, Gudex C, *et al. Statistical projections and scenario forecasts of the adult British: endstage renal failure programme.* A study by the Renal Association and the York Institute of Health Economics (in press).

7 | New drugs for old

Michael D Rawlins
Wolfson Unit of Clinical Pharmacology,
University of Newcastle upon Tyne

Medicines (defined as substances used in the prevention, diagnosis or treatment of disease) have a pivotal role in contemporary clinical practice. Modern vaccines have largely eliminated childhood infectious diseases in the UK such as diphtheria, rubella and poliomyelitis. The appropriate use of antihypertensive agents can reduce significantly the cardiovascular and renal consequences of high blood pressure. Many infections and some cancers can be cured by modern chemotherapeutic agents, and the quality of life of patients suffering from a variety of chronic conditions (including psychiatric, cardiorespiratory, gastrointestinal and dermatological disorders) can be substantially improved with modern drug therapy.

The benefits of modern drugs, however, are obtained only at a price. In 1991, the value of sales of medicines to the National Health Service (NHS) by the pharmaceutical industry was in excess of £3 billion.[1] Over the past ten years the cost of pharmaceutical services in the UK has consistently represented about 10% of total NHS expenditure. With the increasing overall costs of health care delivery, governments, health care planners and managers, and the medical profession itself, have increasingly questioned whether cost savings could be made to the nation's drug bill. In particular, there have been concerns about whether the use of expensive new drugs can be justified on the basis of their cost-effectiveness. This chapter examines what is meant by 'new' drugs, outlines pressures on drug expenditure in both primary and secondary care within the NHS, and considers strategies that might meet current anxieties.

Drug innovation

New pharmaceutical products can best be classified by using a system developed by Lunde and Dukes (Table 1).[2] It is clear from this classification that 'new' drugs form a heterogeneous group of

Table 1. Classification of new pharmaceutical products.[2]

Fully innovative products

1(a) New active substances (new chemical entities or new biological materials) with novel mechanisms of action or fields of application

1(b) Novel pharmaceutical innovations

1(c) Novel combinations used for new purposes

Semi-innovative products

2(a) New active substances belonging to existing therapeutic groups

2(b) Minor pharmaceutical innovations

2(c) Useful fixed-dose combinations of existing drugs

Non-innovative products

3(a) New brands of existing drugs

3(b) Additional preparations of existing drugs (including new dose forms or strengths)

3(c) Traditional combination products

recently introduced pharmaceutical products. New active substances are represented by those in categories 1(a) and 2(a).

Table 2, however, indicates that new active substances represent only a small proportion of new introductions to the pharmaceutical market during an 18-month period in 1991–92, as described in the Monthly Index of Medical Specialties (MIMS).[3] Whilst the numbers in Table 2 will not include all new products launched during the period (non-branded 'generic' products, for example, may not be included in MIMS), the data emphasise the fact that most new products fall within the non-innovative category. Their importance, however, should not necessarily be dismissed. Additional presentations or dosage strengths, for example, may offer significant benefits in relation to patient convenience, and new

Table 2. New product introductions to the UK market in an 18-month period during 1991–92.[3]

Lunde-Dukes category	Innovative category		
	Fully	Semi-	Non-
1	15	34	7
2	0	2	128
3	0	2	7

brands are often cheaper than the market leader. New drugs, in their totality, do not therefore necessarily mean increased costs, and they may bring price competition.

The costs of drug development, which are estimated to be in excess of £70–100 million for a new active substance, mean that new products in Lunde-Dukes classes 1(a) and 2(a) are likely to be significantly more expensive than existing agents. Fully innovative new active substances (Lunde-Dukes class 1(a)) often represent important pharmacological or therapeutic advances. Of the 15 shown in Table 2, seven were new chemical entities and eight new biological or biotechnological products (Table 3). The latter include two *Haemophilus influenzae* B vaccines with major potential public health significance, as well as novel cytokines (filgrastim and molgramostim) for use in relatively small numbers of patients.

The 34 semi-innovative (Lunde-Dukes class 2(a)) products introduced during the same period contrast significantly with the fully innovative products. First, no semi-innovative biotechnological products were brought to the market during this time, emphasising the relatively recent emergence of such agents. Second, the 34 new chemical entities will, by definition, be members of existing pharmacological/therapeutic groups. Their manufacturers will have produced evidence of their efficacy and safety sufficient to satisfy the licensing authority, on the advice of the Committee on

Table 3. Some fully innovatory new active substances introduced during an 18-month period in 1991–92.

	Approved name	Proprietary name
New chemical agents	Adenosine	Adenocor
	Calcipotriol	Dovonex
	Colfosceril	Exosurf
	Finasteride	Proscar
	Halofantrine	Halfan
	Lamotrigine	Lamictal
	Mifepristone	Mifegyne
New biological/ biotechnological agents	Aldesleukin	Proleukin
	Botulinum toxin	Dysport
	Filgrastim	Neupogen
	HA-1A	Centoxin
	Haemophilus influenzae B vaccine	ACT-Hib; Hibtitre
	Hepatitis A vaccine	Havrix
	Molgramostim	Leucomax

Safety of Medicines, to grant product licences for each. Under both domestic (Medicines Act) and European (European Directive 65/65) legislation, however, the licensing authority (and hence the Committee on Safety of Medicines) is specifically excluded from considering comparative efficacy (though *not* comparative safety) when determining licence applications. Consequently, the cost-benefit performance of such products in the context of their use within the NHS may demand further evaluation. On the other hand, the availability of an increased number of similar products provides a potential opportunity for price competition which may be a stimulus for reduced costs.

Prescribing in primary care

The total cost of drugs prescribed in England by doctors in primary health care in 1991–92 was £3.013 billion.[4] This represents a 13.5% increase on the drugs bill in 1990–91.[5] Within the UK, as in most other developed countries, there are thus increasing attempts to control drug costs. Table 4 shows the percentage changes in prescription volume and cost for selected therapeutic classes for the first six months of the 1992–93 financial year compared with 1991–92 in the Northern Region. Within some therapeutic classes (central nervous and respiratory systems) the increase in costs substantially exceeds the increase in volume. This is largely due to the adoption by general practitioners (GPs) of new antidepressants (e.g. selective serotonin reuptake inhibitors) and new bronchodilators (e.g. salmeterol), and the wider use of inhaled steroids in the management of asthma. By contrast, the disproportionate increase

Table 4. Trends (percentage change) in prescription volumes and costs for selected therapeutic classes for 1992–93 compared with 1991–92.

Therapeutic class	Volume (per prescribing unit)	Cost (per prescription)
Central nervous system	+3.9	+13.3
Cardiovascular	+5.1	+2.0
Respiratory	+5.7	+10.3
Gastrointestinal	+6.9	+8.6
Endocrine	+13.2	+3.6
Infections	+3.8	+5.6
Musculoskeletal	+3.2	−1.4

Source: Northern Regional Drug and Therapeutic Centre

in volume of endocrine drugs can be attributed to the wider prescription of relatively inexpensive hormone replacement therapy (HRT). Moreover, the modest (+3.2%) increase in volume of drugs to treat musculoskeletal disorders (mainly non-steroidal anti-inflammatory products) has been accompanied by a slight reduction (–1.4%) in the cost per prescription, perhaps reflecting true price competition in an area where there have been few innovations in recent years.

Secular prescribing changes in primary health care are thus multifactorial. These include the substitution of new drugs for old (e.g. selective serotonin reuptake inhibitors for tricyclic antidepressants), the availability of effective new technologies (e.g. proton pump inhibitors for reflux oesophagitis), and changing therapeutic practice (e.g. inhaled steroids for asthma, or HRT). In such circumstances, conventional concepts of rationing are difficult to apply, and rather different strategies need to be developed in the management of the primary health care budget. First, a research agenda should be developed within the NHS that addresses the pattern and cost-effectiveness of prescribing in general practice, and attempts made to define what good prescribing might look like in a primary health care setting. This would then provide GPs with prescribing standards against which they can judge their own practice.[6]

Second, it is incumbent upon the NHS to encourage comparative studies of the effectiveness of new therapeutic strategies against established ones. This, of course, is merely part of the wider issue of the health technology assessment that is now critically important if the best use is to be made of the resources at our disposal. It also relates to the increasing use of existing technologies as well as the adoption of new ones.

Third, there needs to be a sea change in attitudes to prescribing. The traditional approach to the teaching of therapeutics has been too didactic. Excessive dependence has thus been placed on the views of what are called 'opinion leaders' and 'opinion formers', and too little action taken to ensure that future prescribers understand the significance of clinical trials and assessment of new technologies. We need to ensure that graduates and postgraduates are better able to make their own rational prescribing decisions, based on the results of published scientific evidence.

Prescribing in secondary health care

Although hospital prescribing costs may represent only about 15%

of the total NHS expenditure on drugs, they have a disproportionate effect on the NHS. There is a strong suspicion that, at least in some therapeutic areas, hospital prescribing practice has a significant influence on drug use in primary health care prescribing. Furthermore, the costs of individual products used in hospital may be so great as to distort a hospital's finances and thereby impose restrictions on its other activities. Total drug costs of up to £20,000 per patient per annum are by no means unknown, and may be significantly higher in special circumstances.

Financial pressures on hospital budgets, particularly for high cost/low volume products, have two main origins. They arise either from the increased use of established products or from the adoption of new ones. The further development of a hospital's organ transplantation programme, for example, or the administration of antiviral therapy at an earlier stage of human immunodeficiency virus (HIV) infection, with consequential increase in the use of immunosuppressant or antiviral agents, respectively, may impose major financial strains. Similarly, the introduction of new treatment schedules in the management of specific malignant diseases may have far-reaching consequences for an institution's finances. The rapid introduction of new high cost/low volume products may have even greater financial consequences for major tertiary referral centres.

The control of a hospital's drug expenditure relies on constructive dialogue between its clinicians, pharmacists and managers, in which the hospital's drug and therapeutics committee plays an essential role. Such committees retain the support and confidence of the institution at large only when their efforts to restrict drug costs are accompanied by efforts to encourage good prescribing and to facilitate the introduction of important major therapeutic advances. The strategy for cost containment of low cost/high volume products that I, as Chairman of the Drug and Therapeutics Committee, developed in Newcastle has four features.

Enumeration of true costs

The first part of the strategy, the enumeration of true costs, involves determining the cost of the product for the various categories of patients likely to receive it. It also includes an attempt to obtain estimates of the consequential non-drug costs, such as the need for additional investigations (e.g. plasma drug level measurements) or hospitalisation. In addition, it requires identification of compensatory drug and non-drug savings.

Enumeration of benefits

There is a need to identify a drug's clinical benefits in relation both
to its efficacy and to its safety, and also in comparison with alternative therapeutic strategies currently available. This sometimes
involves at least qualitative, if not quantitative, attempts to determine the effect of the product on patients' quality of life.

Prioritisation of patients

Several categories of patients might be expected to be the benefi-
ciaries for most new products. In such circumstances, it is usually
helpful to obtain a consensus on the various priorities from the relevant clinical specialists. My clinical colleagues invariably take a
highly constructive approach to this difficult and potentially contentious issue, and never fail to reach an agreement—even though
it sometimes involves a remarkable degree of compromise between
them.

Discussions with managers and purchasers

A dialogue with health care managers and purchasers about the
introduction of high cost/low volume new products needs to start
early in the financial planning cycle. The expectation that significant additional resources can be readily identified during the course
of a financial year is illusory. Discussions need to concentrate on
explaining the clinical issues at stake, producing realistic estimates
of the financial consequences, outlining the anticipated 'health
gain', and explaining the basis for the prioritisation of patients.

The strategy outlined above appears to be broadly acceptable to
clinical and managerial colleagues alike. Whilst I am inquisitorial
in my dealings with clinical colleagues, I am their advocate in discussions with managers and purchasers. However, the strategy is
seriously flawed. Although I believe that its principles are substantially correct, the available techniques are too crude for a robust
and reliable quantitative assessment of the impact of new technologies for several reasons:

- financial data within the NHS are too imperfect to give reliable
  estimates of non-drug costs and savings;
- valid measures of the quality of life are unavailable for the purpose of comparative cost-effectiveness;
- prioritisation depends almost exclusively on the judgement of

colleagues rather than on quantitative measures of health gain;
- it is seldom possible to make proactive decisions.

There is an obvious and urgent need within the NHS to develop methods for the evaluation of new technologies which encompass both clinical and economic issues.

Conclusions

Health care systems in all developed countries are facing unprecedented pressures. All countries are seeking ways to reduce health care costs, partly because of demographic trends and partly because of the emergence of new health technologies. Drug budgets will inevitably form part of this scrutiny, and it must be accepted that this will involve a re-examination of some of our current products as well as a more detailed assessment of new ones.

References

1. Association of the British Pharmaceutical Industry. *Annual review 1991–92*. London: ABPI, 1992.
2. Lunde I, Dukes MNG. Les répercussions de la contrôle administrative des médicaments: étude comparée de la situation en Norvège et aux Pays-Bas. *Industrie-Santé* 1980: **49:** 37–57.
3. *Monthly Index of Medical Specialties.* London: Haymarket Medical Ltd.
4. Prescription Pricing Authority. *Annual report 1991–92*. Newcastle upon Tyne: PPA, 1992.
5. Prescription Pricing Authority. *Annual report 1990–91*. Newcastle upon Tyne: PPA, 1992.
6. Department of Health. *Improving prescribing*. London: Department of Health, 1990.

8 | Rationality and rationing: diffused or concentrated decision making?

Rudolf Klein

Professor of Social Policy and Director of the Centre for the Analysis of Social Policy, School of Social Sciences, University of Bath

The starting point for this chapter is a survey carried out recently at Bath into the purchasing plans of health authorities. This was the first stage of a longer-term study, funded by the Nuffield Provincial Hospitals Trust, designed to look at the way in which resource allocation decisions are being taken in the post-1989 National Health Service (NHS). One conclusion stood out from an analysis of the 1992–93 purchasing plans of 114 health authorities: that the radical changes in the structure of the NHS have yet to be translated into equally radical changes in the way health authorities determine their resource allocation policies.[1]

The intention of the purchaser/provider split is that health authorities should determine their resource allocation in the light not of the inherited pattern of services but of the needs of the population. The logic of the split is therefore to push them towards making explicit decisions: to write contracts which specify what services should be provided and in what quantity. In turn, this would seem to imply decisions about rationing, a complex notion which at this stage of the argument will simply be taken to mean determining priorities as between different claims on limited resources.

In practice, the survey suggests, health authorities have been reluctant to choose. Their reaction, when faced with competing claims, has generally been to spread the money around. On average, each purchaser funds 15 priorities, with relatively small amounts often going to each priority. Moreover, it is extraordinarily difficult to winkle out the implications of decisions about resources for the availability of specific services to the population. Very few purchasing plans allow the reader to relate these decisions to any benchmarks of adequacy or need. Lastly, there is little evidence of rationing in the sense of explicitly limiting or denying particular services. Only 12 of the 114 health authorities stated that they would either not buy or limit the availability of specific forms of treatment. Tattoo removal (mentioned by seven health authorities) heads this list, followed by gamete intrafallopian transfer (GIFT)/*in vitro* fertilisation (IVF) (six health authorities). Other forms of treatment or procedures mentioned include adult bat ears, breast augmentation and buttock lift. Clearly, this is rationing at the margins, dealing with the 'small change' of NHS expenditure. These decisions represent symbolic gestures about the need to prioritise between different claims on resources rather than a serious attempt to address the issues. Overall, the purchasing plans represent a commitment to the *status quo*, with the allocation of funds following the existing pattern of spending distribution on services.

How are these findings to be interpreted? One obvious reaction is to say that these are early days, and it is far too soon to expect health authorities to change either their traditional ways of allocating resources or the inherited configuration of services. Certainly, their caution reflects that of the Department of Health, which has been anxious to minimise turbulence and to limit the impact of change on individual providers. The purchasing plans contain at least some hints that health authorities may be bolder in years to come as they gain in experience of the new system and as resource constraints get tighter. However, the survey suggests that there may also be other obstacles in the way of moving towards a more transparent, explicit system for allocating resources and rationing. This chapter therefore explores the conceptual and organisational obstacles likely to be encountered in moving forward. Its theme is that the practice of rationing is inherently difficult, and that progress is therefore likely to be slow and halting. Its aim is to identify the problems involved in the 'search for sunlight'—to quote the editor of the *British Medical Journal*[2]—and to argue that we may have to settle for twilight for some time to come.

The dimensions of rationing

Rationing is a complex and contested notion which needs unpackaging. In ordinary usage, it simply means allocating shares in any given bundle of resources. Thus, the Oxford English Dictionary gives, as an example of an early (1727) use of the term, 'the daily allowance of forage or provender assigned to each horse or other animal'. Implicit in the term, therefore, is some idea of appropriateness or equity, of treating everyone alike according to some defensible criteria, be they horses or human beings. As the common root of the two words would suggest, rationing is closely linked to rationality. To invoke the concept of rationing implies the use of reason in determining the allocation of resources: the sense that, if these resources are limited, the way in which they are distributed to individuals should not be arbitrary but justifiable by appeal to some principles.

However, in the context of the NHS, it is also helpful to think of rationing in terms of a hierarchy of decision-making—where macro-decisions at one level will determine the parameters in which micro-decisions are taken at the next levels. In effect, there are five levels or dimensions of rationing (or resource allocation) in the NHS. They involve decisions about:

1. The size of the total NHS budget, which of course constrains all other subsequent decisions.
2. The allocation of resources to broad sectors or client groups, which may be defined demographically (the elderly) or by the nature of their needs (those suffering from heart disease).
3. The allocation of resources to specific forms of organisational provision (hospital or community?) and treatment (should we invest in new coronary care units?) within such broad categories.
4. The priority to be given to particular types of patients when determining access to the available services and facilities.
5. The level of service to be provided to individual patients once access has been achieved, which may involve choices about either the number of diagnostic procedures to carry out (clinical decisions) or the range of the hotel comforts to be provided (managerial decisions).

Simply to list these difficult levels in the hierarchy of rationing is to underline the complexity of the task faced by health authorities. Decisions about the budgetary allocation to the NHS are clearly outside their scope but constrain all their activities. Decisions about the allocation of funds to particular sectors or groups may be affected by national policy directives but will also be taken by health authorities. Decisions about how much to spend on specific forms of organisational provision or forms of treatment are quintessentially their responsibility. Decisions about how to prioritise access to services has traditionally been left to clinicians, but whether they should be so left in future is, of course, an open question. Decisions about the 'depth' of resources to be devoted to individual patients are very much the responsibility of clinicians, insofar as the use of diagnostic and other services is concerned (though the opposite is true of hotel services).

In a sense, health authorities are caught between two millstones. On the one hand, there are the top-down constraints and priorities and, on the other, the bottom-up pressures. Health authorities face considerable uncertainty about how any given decision about organisational provision and forms of treatment will be translated into practice by clinicians and other health providers. It is a familiar problem when it comes to questions of policy implementation.[3] In framing their policies for resource allocation, health authorities thus face considerable organisational problems. The next section therefore looks at their purchasing policies from the perspective of organisational decision making. If at present their resource allocation policies appear to fall well short of the ideal rationing model—if their purchasing plans lack transparency, coherence and explicit criteria—is this because of some organisational deficiency or because the model demands more than they can be expected to deliver? Could it be that the wrong model is being used to assess their performance?

Models of decision making

Two models dominate the literature on organisational decision making.[4] Both are 'ideal-type' models, and therefore simplify the complex reality, but they provide a useful starting point for discussing the purchasing policies of organisations like health authorities. The first is the *rational, synoptic model*. This conceptualises the organisation rather like a giant computer which comprehensively analyses a problem, searches out all the relevant information and examines the various possible options. It is based on the assumption that there is some optimal solution, usually (though not necessarily) based on a utilitarian type calculus designed to maximise social or organisational benefits. The second is the *incremental model*. This conceptualises the organisation as a coalition of different interests in which decisions will be the outcome of bargaining between those involved and the result of partisan mutual adjustment.

The models can be used either descriptively or prescriptively. Descriptively, the incremental model clearly wins out: muddling through—a policy of incremental adjustments at the edges—tends to be the norm. It certainly describes the purchasing activities of health authorities accurately enough. Prescriptively, however, the rational, synoptic model seems—at first sight—to be more persuasive. Who, after all, can resist the 'rational' label? Who would argue that the process of resource allocation should be based on bargaining or partisan mutual adjustment? In fact, there are good reasons for arguing that the incremental model is not only descriptively but also prescriptively superior to its synoptic rival, and that it is more rational. These arguments rest on the nature of organisational knowledge. If there were no problems about collecting adequate information, scanning all the possible options and analysing the costs and benefits, the giant computer would win hands down. But if there are formidable problems on all these counts, as there are in all organisations, the case for the incremental model of rational decision making becomes that much more persuasive. It is a case for parcelling out and diffusing the task of decision making, making use of information and knowledge scattered through the various levels and professional hierarchies of the organisation. The process of bargaining seen from this perspective is a way of eliciting information, testing options and searching out the most acceptable solution—particularly if it is assumed, contrary to the synoptic model, that there is no one generally accepted currency of evaluation.

Application of models to the health authorities

So much for the theoretical considerations. Applying them to health authorities and to the question of resource allocation is instructive. Consider the issue of information. Despite the proliferation of performance indicators, and the investment in information systems following the NHS reforms, there are still remarkably wide swathes of ignorance. Most conspicuously, it is generally accepted that knowledge is lacking about the outcomes—and therefore the effectiveness—of different interventions or patterns of service provision. Thus, it has been estimated that only about 15% of medical interventions are supported by solid scientific evidence.[5] Much of the information currently available about outcomes or effectiveness is the product not of clinical trials but of clinical experience—a much 'softer' form of knowledge but one which, by definition, is scattered through the organisation.

It may be that, eventually, an investment in outcomes research and clinical trials will help to drain this bog of ignorance, that we will be in a position to assess the outcomes and effectiveness of procedures before introducing them. There are, however, reasons for doubting this; for example, the effectiveness of new techniques will improve as experience increases, thus introducing further

complications into the process of evaluation.[6] Testing the effectiveness of different forms of service provision, as distinct from particular forms of medical intervention, is an even more difficult task.
But, even making heroically optimistic assumptions about the rate
of progress, it may well be a decade or more before health authorities possess all the information required by the synoptic model of
decision making. On less optimistic assumptions, of course, they
will always have to take their decisions on the basis of incomplete
and inadequate information.

The health authorities face equally difficult problems with the
currency used for assessing different options. What currency
would allow them to determine whether priority in the allocation
of resources should be given to services for the elderly as against
services for the mentally handicapped? The problems do not
cease when it comes to deciding priorities between different procedures. On the face of it, quality-adjusted life year (QALY) type
analyses should be able to demonstrate which interventions produce the best yields in terms of the ratio between costs and gains
in health, measured on a common denominator of QALYs. But,
notoriously, there are difficulties about this approach: it assumes
knowledge about outcomes, and is based on a method of 'weighting' different health states that makes strong assumptions about
the ability of interviewers to elicit accurate information both
about people's preferences and about the validity of drawing general conclusions from what are often small samples. Even if
QALY-type calculations are taken at face value, there remains the
question of how far a utilitarian calculus should determine decisions about rationing. Any health service, and perhaps the NHS
in particular, has a symbolic role in society. It is a demonstration
of society's willingness to care, even if this means spending
money on interventions to save lives that could yield a higher
return if spent on chiropody.

There is further difficulty, illustrated by the Oregon version of
the QALY approach.[7] As is well known, this involved ranking different diagnosis–treatment pairs, which, of course, raises the problem of patient heterogeneity: the fact that, within any group, there
will be different responses to intervention (and that, therefore, the
cost-benefit equation will show different results). Hence, the
argument for continuing to delegate rationing decisions of types 4
and 5 to clinicians. As David Mechanic, a distinguished American
medical sociologist, has argued:

> Because patient populations are heterogeneous, many medical inter-
> ventions involve uncertainty, and the clinical decision making process

is iterative (using information obtained from the relationship between professional and patient), an effective health care rationing system must take into account the need for flexible physician response to numerous unprovided-for circumstances. Implicit rationing allows for needed sensitivity to variance by relying on clinical discretion, thus strengthening the potential for professional/patient interaction and making the unwarranted withholding of efficacious services less likely.[8]

This conclusion is reinforced by the experience of many of the health authorities which have sought to adopt a rationing by exclusion approach. In quite a few cases, as the survey showed, the outcome has been a retreat by the authorities concerned. Faced by protests from clinicians, they have concluded that the procedures will not be denied if there is a good clinical case for carrying them out. In short, the decision has passed back to the clinicians concerned. Similarly, even authorities which have sought to adopt a systematic approach to the problem of resource allocation have had to admit bafflement. The main lessons drawn from one such exercise were that there are no easy answers, evidence and information are patchy, it is difficult to do more than change at the margins, and measuring need is hard and complex.[9]

Implications

The analysis presented above suggests that there are two models for taking decisions about rationing—first cousins, as it were, of the two organisational decision models discussed above. The first is what might be styled a *technological model.* Here, the assumption is that, given more information about outcomes, effectiveness, etc., it will be possible to derive priorities almost automatically from the data. The information will speak for itself, provided that the computer is properly programmed. It is a model which would allow top-down decision making by the purchasing authorities.

The second is what might be called a *dialectic model.* Here, the assumption is that information will always be incomplete, and there will always be different views about the criteria to be used in evaluating it. It is a model which allows diffused decision making, and which sees priorities emerging from a process of argument.

The first model depends on technological rationality, and puts the emphasis on more research and the development of better expertise. The second is based on process rationality, and puts the emphasis on improving access to the network of those engaged in debate. If the metaphor for the first is a giant computer, that for the second is a battery of linked personal computers.

Whatever our views about the relative plausibility of the two models, it would seem clear that the conditions for the first model to operate do not as yet exist. Indeed, some would argue, like myself, that they will never exist. So, for the time being at any rate, it would seem that health authorities will have to operate the second model: that is to generate information by parcelling out decision making among different actors, and to see rationing as a process of bargaining, based on a continuing debate about what criteria should be used in making judgements. From this perspective, the apparent unwillingness of health authorities to make hard decisions between competing claims on resources—so far at least—is a sensible response to the problem of inadequate information and uncertainty about the impact of decisions on patients, potential and actual. The most that can be expected is a policy of 'purposeful opportunism', exploiting opportunities as they arise to move in a desired direction.[10]

This is to argue for a policy of incremental and diffused decision making. Decisions about broad priorities (of types 1 to 3) clearly have to be taken by health authorities but, within the constraints imposed by such decisions, it would seem sensible to leave it to clinicians to determine which patients should be treated and how. This conclusion needs to be qualified in one important respect, however. The whole notion of rationing, as suggested earlier, implies allocative decisions based on some explicit and defensible criteria of equity or need. If this point is accepted, this would suggest that clinicians will in turn have to justify the criteria used in their rationing decisions. So, for example, the Dutch Committee on Choices in Health Care has proposed that positions on waiting lists should be decided on the basis of explicit criteria.[11]

In short, just as health authorities have to be accountable for their decisions about resource priorities—in the sense of having to justify the principles which guide their decisions—so clinicians may have to do the same. In the past, they have been reluctant to do so. Clinical autonomy has been translated to mean lack of explicit criteria against which to judge the performance of those entrusted with using public resources. In future, it may be to the advantage of the medical profession to change this stance. Public knowledge about how resources are being used at the point of delivery—the fourth and fifth dimensions of rationing—would also allow some judgement to be made about the adequacy or otherwise of the initial rationing decision which constrains all others: that made by the government when determining the budget of the NHS.

References

1. Klein R, Redmayne S. *Patterns of priorities*. Birmingham: National Association of Health Authorities and Trusts, 1992.
2. Smith R. Rationing: the search for sunlight. *British Medical Journal* 1991; **303**: 1561–2.
3. Lipsky M. *Street-level bureaucracy*. New York: Russell Sage Foundation, 1980.
4. Braybrooke D, Lindblom CE. *A strategy of decision*. New York: The Free Press, 1963.
5. Smith R. Where is the wisdom . . ? *British Medical Journal* 1991; **303**: 798–9.
6. Jennett B. *High technology medicine*. Oxford: Oxford University Press, 1986.
7. Klein R. Warning signals from Oregon. *British Medical Journal* 1992; **304**: 1457–8.
8. Mechanic D. Professional judgment and the rationing of medical care. *University of Pennsylvania Law Review* 1992; **140**: 1713–54.
9. Heginbotham C, Ham C. *Purchasing dilemmas*. London: King's Fund College, 1992.
10. Klein R, O'Higgins M. Social policy after incrementalism. In: Klein R, O'Higgins M, eds. *The future of welfare*. Oxford: Basil Blackwell, 1985.
11. Dunning AJ (chairman). *Report of the Government Committee on Choices in Health Care*. Rijswijk, Netherlands: Ministry of Welfare, Health and Cultural Affairs, 1992.

9 | The district health authority decision process

Jack Howell
*Chairman, Southampton and
South West Hampshire Health Authority, and
Emeritus Professor of Medicine, University of Southampton*

Ever since the National Health Service (NHS) began, demands for care have continually exceeded the capacity of the service to provide it. Overexpenditure has been a regular phenomenon and, until about 1980, additional resources were provided at an average rate of 4% per annum to meet the deficit and to finance some new developments. For about the next six years, the average increase provided each year was reduced to about 1%, and the excess expenditure was no longer made good—that is, the health service was now cash-limited (Fig. 1).

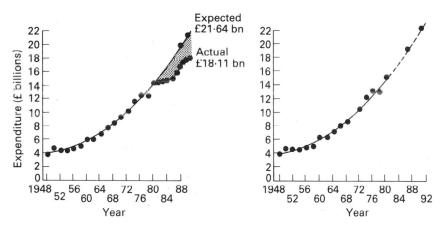

Fig. 1. *Changes in National Health Service funding before and after 1980–81.*[1] (a) Expenditure on NHS in England 1948–80 corrected to 1986 prices by annual retail price index. Best fit curve is extrapolated to show expenditure expected if annual rate of increase (4% compound) had been maintained. Between 1980 and 1986, rate of increase slowed to about 1% (shaded area: gap between expected and actual expenditure); (b) after 1986, rate of increase was increased substantially, but a gap of about £0.5 bn per annum remained in 1990. (Reproduced with permission from Ref. 1)

The financial pressures resulting from this lower rate of growth of funding were expected to be met by improved efficiency. Despite the major reorganisation of the NHS in 1982, and the introduction of general management in 1985, the improvements in efficiency were insufficient to make up for the reduced rate of increase in funding. In many areas, there was difficulty in providing care to all who needed it. Politically embarrassing crises continued to occur until they precipitated the Prime Ministerial Review and the NHS and Community Care Act of 1990.

Since 1991, the NHS has been working under these reforms which made the radical change of separating the functions of purchasing and providing health care. The development of independent provider trusts within the NHS has been encouraged and widely adopted, with the result that these separate functions are increasingly carried out by separate organisations—district health authorities (DHAs) as purchasers, and the hospital and community trusts as providers.

The reforms have been directed at the more efficient and more effective use of resources, so that the original objective of the NHS of providing a comprehensive health service available to all would continue to be met. The term 'comprehensive' is defined in the Oxford English Dictionary as 'comprising much; of large content or scope'. It does not mean all-embracing.

This chapter will describe the way in which DHAs make decisions about the purchase of health care for their local population in the context of the possible need to ration health care. My view is that a stage has not been reached at which explicit rationing is inevitable, but the possibility is undoubtedly now very much greater.

Some patients have always been unable to obtain care at the time they need it. There have always been waiting lists, and also some patients in whom the probability of benefit has been so low that clinicians have decided or were prepared not to offer treatment. Most health care could be provided, but perhaps not some care at the margins. The bases of these decisions were not made explicit, and hence this is sometimes referred to as implicit rationing.

The question today is whether the stage has been reached at which it is inevitable that we must be explicit in deciding that some patients who would benefit will be denied care and, if so, by whom and by what process.

Nothing in the new NHS Act provides more resources directly. The Act has provided a framework within which it is possible to identify more clearly what is being done and how and, hopefully, to see ways of providing care most efficiently and effectively. If this process is successful, it will be possible to provide a greater amount of care and at least postpone the need for explicit rationing. I have long thought, perhaps overoptimistically, that if government were confident that the resources were being used efficiently, they would be more likely to allocate more.

The decision process in district health authorities

Before April 1991, when the Act was implemented, the majority of health care demands were already being met, so planning did not have to start from scratch. To ensure that disruption of the service was minimised with the introduction of the new system in April 1991, DHAs were instructed to do the same in 1991–92 as they had in 1989–90 (the last year for which full data were available).

This care was to be specified in terms of activities and costs—as 'service agreements' or contracts. Three types of contract were possible:

- block contracts;
- costs and volume contracts;
- cost per case contracts.

Specification of the clinical content of the block contracts was limited. Experience in this first year began to provide the database for contracting in the succeeding years when modifications to these contracts might be required.

Southampton and South West Hampshire District Health Authority

While the overall process was common to all Districts, the detailed implementation differed because of variations in local circumstances and local problems. In the Southampton and South West Hampshire Health Authority the majority of services were allocated under block contracts, and covered most of the needs. There were exceptions: some services, such as pacemaker implants and termination of pregnancy, were covered by cost and volume contracts with certain providers.

The validity of much of the data on which the contracts were placed was tested in this first year, and improvements began to be made, but this is only a beginning. Some financial adjustments were often necessary during the year, but perhaps the most important lesson from this first year was that provider units no longer had the option of dealing with financial crises by reducing services, for example closing wards, because the activity to be achieved had been agreed in the contract.

Table 1. Procedures not purchased by Southampton and South West Hampshire District Health Authority (1991–92).

- *In vitro* fertilisation/donor insemination
- Cosmetic plastic surgery
- Reversals of sterilisation
- Asymptomatic wisdom teeth
- Tattoo removal
- Asymptomatic varicose veins
- Certain orthopaedic procedures

In recognition of the pressures on resources, the DHA has made some attempts to limit the range of care available by denying certain patients access to some services, but quantitatively the effect is very small (Table 1). These exclusions largely refer to disorders for which few doctors would give these treatments priority, given the current pressures on resources. The main purpose of these exclusions is to prevent such patients being put on to the waiting lists and distorting priorities, now that maximum waiting times have been defined. An exclusion made for different reasons, however, is *in vitro* fertilisation. Several years ago, after much debate, the Southampton DHA reluctantly decided that this was of lower priority compared with other demands on resources. It was a carefully considered decision by the DHA, reflecting its first responsibility, which is to the whole of the community to make the best use of the resources provided to it.

Better use of resources

No DHA would wish to extend its list of exclusions rather than promote the better use of resources by its providers, so what can DHAs do to achieve this?

First, a DHA must manage its purchasing function with efficiency. It must negotiate good agreements with providers, and not be generous or profligate with its money (this should go without saying). The possibility of placing contracts with other providers increases its influence in this process of negotiation with providers. In a district like Southampton, where there is a limited number of potential providers for patients in whom speed of access is important, the ability to choose alternative providers is also limited, but there are many areas of elective care where speed of access is not important. Patients are often prepared to travel to other districts if treatment there can be offered more quickly. This helps in negotiating the provision of care at lower cost consistent with the preservation of standards of quality.

Second, DHAs need advice on what should be purchased for their local community, and they need to discuss carefully with providers better ways of providing care. Both purchasers and providers have this as a common objective—this is their *raison d'être*—but the interests of the two organisations may of course differ when the contracts to provide care are being hammered out. While the DHA specifies the quantity and quality of care and, where possible, the expected outcomes, it is largely for the provider, not the purchaser, to decide the best way of achieving the aims of the contract, and thereby offer the best contract to potential purchasers. Providers have an incentive to be efficient.

The point to make here is that the purchaser/provider separation, for all the immediate problems that this may create, can lead to better use of resources and thereby prevent or delay the need to accept the necessity of explicit rationing of care.

Meeting the demand for health care within available resources

It is recognised that this system may impose great responsibility on the provider units, especially if they have difficulty in meeting the requirements of the contracts. Unless the DHA is explicit in which care it will not purchase, responsibility for choosing which patients shall receive care remains, as previously, with the clinicians, the doctors and the nurses, and this can be a hard and difficult process. The DHA recognises the dilemma for provider units of having greater demand for care than can readily be met within the resources available, and that it can be resolved in only a limited number of ways:

- by choosing not to treat certain individuals, on grounds of poor likelihood of benefit, or higher cost in relation to benefit in the broadest sense;
- by recognising that some forms of care are ineffective, and thereby discontinuing them, for example, some forms of heroic surgery with poor prognosis;
- by employing cheaper but equally effective strategies of care, for example day surgery in place of inpatient care, or developing agreed protocols for care—this is an area where prior discussion between the DHA and providers leading to specification in the contract is likely to influence the way in which care is delivered more cheaply and effectively;

- by compromising on quality, for example by choosing cheaper drugs with less benefit, shorter durations of stay than are optimal, etc.—but this would be contrary to the contract agreement;
- by the use of more efficient administrative and secretarial methods, for example shifting resources within clinical directorates from non-patient work to be available for patient care.

The final resort is explicit rationing of care—the decision to deny some patients care from which they might benefit by moving the boundary of decision of the probability of benefit and requiring a greater probability. This could be a decision made openly, as in Oregon, or by clinicians who would make such a decision only if they felt it was defensible in the individual case. It would be unacceptable for the clinician to have to make choices that were unequivocally against the best interests of the patient.

The alternative is to have ever-lengthening waiting lists. This has been the traditional way of dealing with the problem: not deciding *whether* to treat, but *when* to treat, recognising that this might be a very long time, possibly never. This, however, is no longer an option, because the maximum time which patients may have to wait has now been limited by a policy decision taken centrally.

Explicit rationing?

Is explicit rationing the next step? My view is that it is to be avoided until there is really no alternative. However, to continue to place responsibility upon the clinician for choosing who will receive care has some worrying consequences. At the heart of the concern is the need to preserve, as far as possible, confidence in the doctor–patient relationship. This is destroyed if the doctor is seen to be, or even suspected of, making decisions which are clearly not in the interests of the patient, but solely in the interest of the best use of resources. How long this professional independence can be preserved depends upon the success of the co-operation between management and the professions in working out more cost-effective procedures.

When this route has been exhausted there would seem to be only two alternatives, either:

- more resources must be provided, which could now be argued for from a position of considerable strength; or
- the need to ration care must be accepted, beginning with some of the less essential forms of care.

District health authority decisions relating to developments in the service

DHAs need to provide for new developments and new services which may sometimes be more desirable than some of the existing services. For example, the DHA may wish to introduce new forms of clinical investigation and treatment, such as fluoridation of the water supply, which is a current priority in Southampton because of the high prevalence of dental decay in our school-children. The DHA may wish to change the balance of primary and secondary care on grounds of economy and patient preference, or perhaps to strengthen health promotion and prevention of disease. How are decisions made about these and where do the resources come from? Some of the issues and problems were explored in a simulation exercise held by Southampton DHA in 1991, called Purchasing Dilemmas, which has been reported in a special publication with the King's Fund College.[2]

Each year, when the DHA has agreed on the contracts (suitably modified) to be let for existing services, it begins to see how much money may be available for such improvements but, before proceeding, the financial implications of a number of other priorities have to be assessed. These priorities are listed in ranking order in Table 2. The last four reflect the need to rank even the local priorities. Given that there is some money remaining after the higher priorities have been met, the DHA must decide what it will purchase in the best interests of the community.

The health commissions

The health commissions are important in making these decisions. Currently there are two statutory bodies: the Family Health Services Authority, responsible for family health services; and the DHA, responsible for the purchase of secondary and community

Table 2. Priority bands for purchasing by Southampton and South West Hampshire District Health Authority (1991–92).

Band 1:	Commitments
Band 2:	National priorities
Band 3:	Regional Health Authority priorities
Band 4:	Highest local priorities
Band 5:	Second highest local priorities
Band 6:	Third highest local priorities
Band 7:	Other local priorities

services. These two authorities are charged with working closely together, but there are many difficulties. Some regions, including Wessex, have overcome this by creating health commissions to provide a single purchasing strategy for primary, secondary and community care. The purchasing decisions of a health commission are therefore more widely based, and require a wider range of information and advice across all these services.

A health commission has to be aware of, and be sensitive to, the views of a wide range of groups:

* the public through the Community Health Councils (CHCs) and other routes;
* the general practitioners (GPs), who are in close touch with the needs of their communities;
* the midwives and nurses.

The Director of Public Health is charged with reporting on the health (and illness) of the district in the annual report, which is another vital source of information to be assimilated and incorporated into the strategy.

In 1992, the Southampton and South West Hampshire Health Commission agreed a purchasing strategy for the next five years. This followed wide consultation with GPs, the CHC, the Medical Advisory Committee of the DHA, nursing and other groups, and provider units. A draft plan was prepared and discussed by the health commission. It was then considered at a public meeting, and eventually accepted as the purchasing strategy for the coming five years. The ultimate decisions about purchasing rest with the health commission, and it is important that they are made following consultation and not prior to it.

Conclusions

The subject of this book is the rationing of medical care. Professor Klein has indicated that his review of the purchasing plans of a large number of DHAs has shown that rationing is not a prominent feature of the contracting process at present, and it is pleasing that he has concluded that this is probably the right approach at the present time. I believe that these decisions may well be looming, but are not yet inevitable. There may be a need to restrict care from time to time on an *ad hoc* basis to meet short-term deficiencies. The time to restrict care by explicit rationing is when existing resources are being optimally, efficiently and effectively used and, despite this, clinicians are having to make decisions which conflict with their ethical principles. Only then need the DHA or health commission consider explicit rationing.

References

1. Re-examining the fundamental principles of the NHS. *British Medical Journal* 1992; **304**: 297–9.
2. *Purchasing dilemmas.* Special report by King's Fund College and Southampton and South West Hampshire Health Authority. London: King's Fund, 1992.

10 | The role of the regional health authority in prioritisation

Bob Nicholls
Chief Executive, Oxford Regional Health Authority

I hope that this final chapter will put into context some of the many other aspects of rationing of health care that have been covered so far and, at this time of speculation about the future of regions, will demonstrate that the regional health authorities (RHAs) do have a part to play in the critically important topic of prioritisation in health care.

Objectives of the Oxford Regional Health Authority

The Oxford RHA has six key objectives, each of which can be seen to have something to do with its role in prioritisation (Table 1). The Region is charged with setting the strategic framework for purchasers of health care. It then:

- backs this framework by distributing resources to the purchasing authorities;
- encourages and monitors the best use of these resources;
- promotes the rights and needs of the individual for health care;
- sets standards and trains staff to deliver; and
- networks and communicates to keep the framework alive.

The role of an RHA may be simply summed up by four key tasks, two of which relate to the regulation of the National Health Service (NHS) managed market:

1. Production of a strategic framework of broad policies and standards to regulate the health care market.
2. Allocation of financial resources.
3. Conciliation and regulation of relationships between authorities.
4. Audit and improvement of authorities' performances.

I will attempt to show how regions' key roles contribute to the process of prioritisation.

Table 1. Objectives of the Oxford Regional Health Authority.

- **Health policies and priorities:**
  Developing a clear health strategy, and working with district and family health service authorities and general practitioner fund-holders to develop purchasing plans and contracts which achieve objectives based on national and regional priorities and local needs.

- **Financial strategy:**
  Allocating funds available to the Region to support these objectives.

- **Value for money:**
  Assisting and encouraging the authorities and National Health Service Trusts to achieve their objectives by utilising their funds in the most efficient and cost-effective way.

- **Patient care:**
  Encouraging authorities and health workers to behave in ways that respect patients as individuals and put their needs first.

- **Leadership:**
  Creating within the Region an environment of mutual respect, trust and commitment to quality, service, excellence and innovation. Within this environment, staff will be encouraged to develop their abilities to the full.

- **Collaboration:**
  Collaborating with other agencies and bodies in the health care and related fields to provide the greatest benefit to the local community.

Allocation of resources in the National Health Service

In his Autumn Statement the Chancellor gave a first indication of the amount of money that the NHS will get in 1993, which allows the Secretary of State for Health and the National Health Service Management Executive (NHSME) to determine the amount of money that each of the 14 RHAs in England and Wales will be given to allocate for the commissioning and provision of health care. Prior to the Statement, several choices will have been made. The government will have decided what overall level of public service spending the country can afford—£244 bn or whatever—and, having listened to the arguments of the competing Ministers of State, the total amount of money to be spent on the NHS in the forthcoming year.

Although the subject under discussion is rationing in medicine, it is important to remember that prioritising and rationing occur at *all* levels of a nation's decision making. Moreover, every time a ranking is made of priorities, the same sort of process occurs.

Complex value judgements involving relative weighting of needs, moral and political judgements, and economic considerations, are made by groups in order to reach decisions.

Once the money has been allocated, the NHS begins another round of prioritising: how much weighting is to be given to general medical services, next year as opposed to hospital and community services, and how much importance will be given to making progress with the recommendations of the Tomlinson Report[1] or other national initiatives? Examples in recent years have included acquired immune deficiency syndrome, Project 2000, Achieving a Balance, and reducing junior doctors' hours, and waiting lists. How much should be reserved for the important caring for people legislation? Finally, how much should be given to each of the 14 RHAs? In the division of resources among the 14 regions, there is the first explicit attempt to formalise the rationing mechanism by trying to assess the relative amount of need for health services that exists in each region. The system works on a weighted capitation basis, taking account of the age of populations and the square root of standardised mortality ratios (SMRs). It attempts a type of equity, not of expenditure but of resource input as defined by this formula.

Two ways of demonstrating the effects of resource distribution policy are the distances the regions are from their Resource Allocation Working Party (RAWP) revenue targets (Fig. 1), and the total NHS net expenditures per person (Table 2).[2]

Resource distribution in the regional health authorities

This same formula, in turn, informs the first set of choices that are made by the RHA, which result in the relative shares allocated to each purchasing district. The method is neither entirely fair nor precise. It can and does lead to possible distortions, for example, the currently observed shift from inner-city areas to more prosperous commuter areas and retirement communities. Regions can put other factors into the formula, including social deprivation and the amount of private hospital care in the health authority areas. Some Regions do this, but Oxford RHA has found such refinements complex, prone to challenge, and marginal in their effect, so has chosen thus far to stick with the national formula. Nonetheless, Oxford RHA too is progressing towards equalisation of its weighted capitation targets (Fig. 2).

The priority issue is the pace towards capitation targets: with low growth, a fast pace will cause serious problems for some purchasers

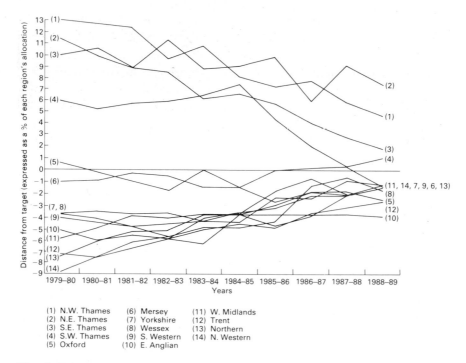

Fig. 1. *Distance of the 14 regional health authorities in England and Wales from their Resource Allocation Working Party targets (1979–89).*(Reproduced with permission of HMSO)

Table 2. Total National Health Service net expenditures per person (excludes centrally financed services).

	1980	1986	1992*	% Change 1980–90†
United Kingdom	162	305	531	1.0
England	151	296	518	0.9
Wales	164	318	560	2.0
Scotland	189	363	619	1.2
Northern Ireland	202	365	606	0.4
Oxford Regional Health Authority	136	247	432	0.7

*Estimated expenditure.
†Figures adjusted by NHS Pay and Price indices in England.
Source: Health and Personal Social Services, Supply Estimates and Government Expenditure Plans.

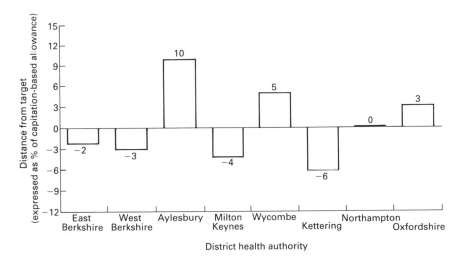

Fig. 2. *Distance of the eight district health authorities in the Oxford Regional Health Authority from their capitation targets: percentage post-1992–93 capitation-based allocations.*

and their providers, but a slow pace will continue to deprive the below target districts. Other problems include the inability always to obtain accurate annual population profiles, and the non-recognition by the method of patterns of services and priorities established during nearly half a century of NHS provision. However, despite some inadequacies, the method is generally recognised as less unfair than other systems.

Establishing the principles of prioritisation at regional level

If this were the only role for the region in prioritising, it would be difficult but relatively short work. What more can and does the RHA do in establishing the principles through which prioritising of health care services occurs? First, it keeps in mind the aim of the health service to balance individual and population needs (Fig. 3). When discussing health services at regional level which, even in a small region, involves a billion pounds, $2\frac{1}{2}$ million people and 50,000 staff, it is easy to forget that the best use of resources is one which finds and then maintains this delicate balance between the health needs of the population and the care and attention to the individual.

Thus far, in using weighted capitation to distribute money, the NHS is operating on the principle of population equity, as far as possible. Allocations have been made in a way that attempts to get

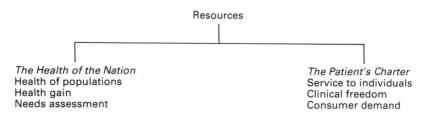

Fig. 3. *The health care balance.*

resources to communities that are roughly equal to the needs of their population as expressed by the formula. The tasks of purchasing authorities, however, may well be unequal because of the relative differences in the historical pattern of health provision in each community and the efficiency with which resources have been used. Also, until recently the allocation of resources for primary care from its separate parliamentary vote was on an entirely different distribution method. This has resulted in very uneven provision of primary care services, again as Sir Bernard Tomlinson's report on London has amply demonstrated.[1]

Having agreed the method by which resources are broadly distributed between the purchasing authorities, the RHAs set national and regional priorities and may well add to the national top slicing, for example, for supporting training, research and development (R&D), or clinical innovation, and by setting aside special strategic or programme funding before finally making allocations to purchasing authorities and to general practitioner fund-holders. It is only then that prioritising health services through purchasing contracts takes place. These contracts often have to be drawn up in the context of guidelines set by the NHSME and the regions to encourage value for money and meet quality guidelines. The regions play a part in all these processes.

First, the regions always look for efficiency savings. The NHS has been asked for efficiency savings for so many years now that it is tempting to think there are no more to be found but, as recent Audit Commission reports have demonstrated, there is still some way to go in most provider units, for example, in day surgery, estate management, bed use, nurse deployment and skill mix, and laboratory services. In a fast-changing world of new health care systems and new techniques, and old ones becoming cheaper or redundant, there will always be opportunities to improve efficiency. This is not just about honing cleaning contracts by competitive scrutiny, but every area of the country has hospitals with inefficient sites, large heating and waste bills, expensive support services, too much paper, duplication of investigations and unnecessary appointments. Generic prescribing in primary care in Oxford Region would save at least an estimated £5 million. Throughout the country there are large numbers of procedures for which day care is clinically appropriate, but which are not performed on a day basis. Are generic prescribing and day care about efficiency? Do these examples impinge on clinical freedom?

It is important that the quest for value for money should continue and broaden, and the region has an important role to play in setting efficiency targets, helping to identify possible areas for review, pump priming, providing examples of good practice, analysing and publishing variations and monitoring results.

Second, the region tries to consider how effective are the health services it delivers. Is it known how much improvement in health will occur from a particular contact with the health services? Can the level of patient satisfaction from a particular procedure be assessed, and how sure are we that the treatment will produce a beneficial outcome?

The Cochrane Centre, the national centre for research into the outcomes of randomised controlled trials, has recently opened in Oxford. By summing the results of randomised controlled trials in the field of pregnancy and childbirth, its Director, Dr Iain Chalmers, has provided conclusively the striking benefits of some procedures and the relative worthlessness and even harm of others;[3] yet not all the beneficial ones are practised, and some of the worthless ones continue to be practised in the UK. While the cost to the NHS of ineffective procedures must be enormous, the outcome to the patient is at best minimal. Conversely, some very effective treatments have been confirmed by this approach. For example, the International Study of Infarct Survival (ISIS) trials have shown that survival after myocardial infarction can be dramatically improved by a combination of streptokinase and aspirin. A lot is still not known, but the application of even a part of what is now known would result in considerably better use of health resources. It is part of the regions' responsibilities to foster the necessary R & D, focused now by the national R & D programmes, and to disseminate the results, challenging purchasers whose plans fail to reflect this type of information.

Third, how good is quality control and risk management in health services? If quality health care is about getting the best possible care commensurate to the need, and about getting it right first time, quality control improves the ability to use the resources in the system well. Is it known how well Hospital A does against Hospital B with regard to infections and re-admissions, or why Hospital A has a better set of outcomes than Hospital B for a given procedure? What can be done to stem the rising tide and cost of medical negligence?

Rationing of services

While I have not yet mentioned rationing of services, I believe that prioritisation is in part about the best use of scarce resources. In each area of efficiency, effectiveness and quality, the RHA has a major role in identifying good practice, promoting it, and ensuring that purchasers take it into account when awarding their contracts.

Nearly two decades ago, the then Minister of Health, Barbara Castle, wrote words that have been pinned on the walls of many a weary health authority manager: 'Choices are difficult, but choose we must'. Ministerial choices may have been difficult, but for many in the NHS the system for many years was quite straightforward. In general, a hospital would expect to get roughly what it already had, with a bit added for inflation, a bit more if it had complained to the right people during the year, and a bit more for any emergencies. Occasionally, there was a lot more for a good development in a priority field or as part of a major capital development.

Yet the simple fact is that the NHS has always prioritised and always rationed, often by individual clinicians using professional judgements to make choices in opaque processes and procedures in GP surgeries, outpatient suites and wards. Similarly, decisions, for example, on capital investment were taken using equally obscure political and bureaucratic processes. These processes are now being stripped of their protective layers and made transparent for all to question. This is not an easy or comfortable process. The RHA has given a certain sum of money to the purchasing authority to buy services for its population. Like the Cabinet several months previously, the purchasing authority will meet and bring a set of individual judgements to match limited resources against needs and demands. The RHA has the responsibility to inform, assess, monitor and generally oversee these purchasing plans.

Models of rationing[d]

Two models of rationing have emerged. The first, famously used in the Oregon project, is to ration by excluding certain types of treatment or conditions from definitions of approved needs. This approach has been so far used by a minority of health authorities in the UK which have said that they will not purchase, for example, tattoo removal, the extraction of wisdom teeth or infertility treatment. Although this method has its attractions, particularly the testing of professional and epidemiological advice against consumer values, it also appears to have a number of weaknesses. The fact that people pick on tattoo removal to illustrate it shows that value judgements are not based on effectiveness but on the acceptability of that type of treatment to people who will never need it, an example of what has been called in America 'bourgeoisie sparing the bourgeoisie'.

It also risks the morally unacceptable practice of excluding certain people from particular treatments, as Professor Grimley Evans has powerfully shown for older people. However, to me the great achievement of the Oregon approach is to get rationing out of the closet and to raise the standard of the public debate. I believe that a similar approach will come to the UK as needs and demands further outstrip supply.

The second rationing method has now become embodied in *The health of the nation* White Paper. This approach rations by identifying the groups within the population who will benefit to the greatest degree. It seeks to achieve the best balance of benefits, risks and costs when using the resources available for health care (Table 3). Here, the RHA must lead by establishing protocols for health purchasing, publishing health outcomes, and ensuring that purchasers are well informed about the choices that confront them.

Oxford Regional Health Authority strategic framework

In April 1991, Oxford RHA took Healthgain, which it explained in shorthand as 'adding life to years, and years to life', as a cornerstone for the regional strategic framework Towards 2000. Together with the three other foundations of value for money, quality, and consumer responsiveness, this set the scene for purchasers beginning the process of commissioning health care. Anticipating *The health of the nation*, Oxford RHA chose six priority healthgain

Table 3. The health gain approach.

- What are the health problems of the population?
- What impact can the National Health Service have?
- What are the priorities?
- What are the desired outcomes?
- How can these be measured?
- What service strategies will achieve these outcomes?

areas and developed these into a set of healthgain protocols to provide advice to purchasers on investment decisions and purchasing plans (Table 4).

Table 4. Oxford Regional Health Authority (RHA) strategic framework Towards 2000.

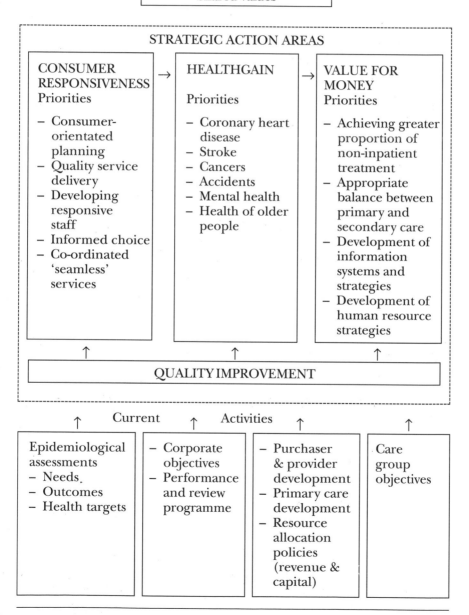

| RHA Mission statement: Shared values |

STRATEGIC ACTION AREAS

CONSUMER RESPONSIVENESS Priorities	→	HEALTHGAIN Priorities	→	VALUE FOR MONEY Priorities
– Consumer-orientated planning – Quality service delivery – Developing responsive staff – Informed choice – Co-ordinated 'seamless' services		– Coronary heart disease – Stroke – Cancers – Accidents – Mental health – Health of older people		– Achieving greater proportion of non-inpatient treatment – Appropriate balance between primary and secondary care – Development of information systems and strategies – Development of human resource strategies

QUALITY IMPROVEMENT

Current   Activities

| Epidemiological assessments
– Needs
– Outcomes
– Health targets | – Corporate objectives
– Performance and review programme | – Purchaser & provider development
– Primary care development
– Resource allocation policies (revenue & capital) | Care group objectives |

Making choices

This process, in the hands of the epidemiologists, sounds beauti-
fully logical and reasonable, until it comes into the cold light of
health services' choices. Consider the national priority of heart disease. A purchaser has so much money allocated for health care in
a district. How should it be spent on health interventions relating
to heart disease? Perhaps the heart surgeons in provider units have
become very efficient and effective at performing coronary artery
bypass grafts (as they have in Oxford), yet purchasers' take-up is
very variable (Table 5).

Perhaps rehabilitation services were promised more finance last
year. They are very popular with patients, but all the statistics show
their effectiveness, as measured by outcomes, is low. The district
health authority might have an SMR below the national average, but
the rate of heart disease in young men is rising significantly, and *The
health of the nation* sets targets for reduction, not absolute targets to
be achieved. A health education programme could target the risk
groups, but its impact is uncertain. Our priority is to save lives and
we do, say the surgeons. Our priority is to add life to years and we
can, say the paramedics. Our priority is to achieve health for all and
we will, say the health promoters—at a better cost per quality-adjusted life year say the health economists. Yet the increase of coronary
heart disease and the demand for effective treatments will continue
to rise. How will purchasing authorities make the priority choices

Table 5. Coronary artery bypass monitoring in the Oxford Regional
Health Authority 1992–93.

Purchaser	Target (300 pmp)	Forecast (1st quarter only)
District:		
1	112	140
2	139	108
3	45	20
4	79	32
5	62	40
6	80	28
7	98	52
8	168	280
Region	783	700

pmp = per million population

between these conflicting and well articulated interests, even within a particular high priority disease group?

Despite the rhetoric, a recent survey by the National Association of Health Authorities and Trusts (NAHAT) indicates that purchasing authorities are not yet very confident about their rationing choices. NAHAT found that, rather than making explicit choices between competing priorities, authorities are preferring to 'spread the money around'. Those few authorities which have chosen to ration by excluding certain categories are generally opting for qualifications: for example, 'the following types of referral outside contract will *probably* be refused' (West Surrey & NE Hampshire, personal communication). This may be a relief to some people; it may also be a reflection of two generous public expenditure rounds. The danger is that what is now a fudge will turn into a mess. If purchasing authorities do not sharpen the tools to allow them to make choices,[5] and the RHAs do not take the sort of lead I have described in providing the tools, they will never be able to think clearly about choices when they have to do so, nor will they be able to account for the decisions they have made.

Conclusions

I have tried to demonstrate that priority choices have to be made at all levels in a service that is still over 80% publicly funded. Before rationing decisions about what services not to provide are taken, it is essential to address efficiency, effectiveness and quality. The debate is not about *whether* to prioritise, but how best to do it. I believe that the separation of responsibility for purchasing and providing health care has provided a framework for the more explicit and objective determination of priorities, and that one or two years of little or no real growth will require the purchasers to make more difficult choices. Regions have a vital role in giving them a framework and tools for this demanding task, challenging the appropriateness of these choices and, if necessary, securing political support for them.

At a time when we in Oxford have been powerfully reminded of Archie Cochrane,[6] and with the Secretary of State battling for an adequate share of an inadequate public sector cake, when thinking of prioritisation we could do worse than to recall one of Cochrane's hypotheses, that all *effective* treatment should be free (i.e. available on the NHS). It will not take us all the way, but it would be a good start and provide a powerful common agenda for politicians, purchasers, providers and professionals.

References

1. *Inquiry into London's health service, medical education and research:* the Tomlinson Report. London: HMSO, 1992.
2. Ham C. *The new National Health Service: organisation and management.* Oxford: National Association of Health Authorities and Trusts, Radcliffe Medical Press, 1990.
3. Chalmers I, ed. *A guide to effective care in pregnancy and childbirth.* Oxford University Press.
4. Dunning AJ (Chairman). *Report of the Government Committee on Choices in Health Care.* Rijswijk, Netherlands: Ministry of Welfare, Health and Cultural Affairs, 1992.
5. *Purchasing dilemmas.* Special report by King's Fund College and Southampton and South West Hampshire District Health Authority. London: King's Fund, 1992.
6. Cochrane A. *Random reflection on health services.* Rock Carling Lecture. London: Nuffield Provincial Hospitals Trust, 1972.